BLUEPR
Pediat
Infectious
Diseases

Blueprints **for your pocket!**

In an effort to answer a need for high yield review books for the elective rotations, Blackwell Publishing now brings you Blueprints in pocket size.

These new Blueprints provide the essential content needed during the shorter rotations. They will also provide the basic content needed for USMLE Steps 2 and 3, or if you were unable to fit in the rotation, these new pocket-sized Blueprints are just what you need.

Each book will focus on the high yield essential content for the most commonly encountered problems of the specialty. Each book features these special appendices:

- Career and residency opportunities
- Commonly prescribed medications
- Self-test Q&A section

Ask for these at your medical bookstore or check them out online at www.blackwellmedstudent.com

Blueprints Dermatology
Blueprints Urology
Blueprints Pediatric Infectious Diseases
Blueprints Ophthalmology
Blueprints Plastic Surgery
Blueprints Orthopedics
Blueprints Hematology and Oncology
Blueprints Anesthesiology
Blueprints Infectious Diseases

BLUEPRINTS
Pediatric
Infectious
Diseases

Samir S. Shah, MD
Instructor, Department of Pediatrics
University of Pennsylvania School of Medicine
Fellow, Divisions of Infectious Diseases and General Pediatrics
The Children's Hospital of Philadelphia
Philadelphia, PA

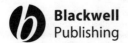

Blackwell
Publishing

Blackwell Publishing, Inc., 350 Main Street, Malden, Massachusetts 02148-5018, USA
Blackwell Publishing Ltd, 9600 Garsington Road, Oxford OX4 2DQ, UK
Blackwell Publishing Asia Pty Ltd, 550 Swanston Street, Carlton, Victoria 3053, Australia

04 05 06 07 5 4 3 2 1

ISBN: 1-4051-0402-3

Library of Congress Cataloging-in-Publication Data

Blueprints pediatric infectious diseases / [edited by] Samir S. Shah.—1st ed.
    p. ; cm. — (Blueprints)
  Includes index.
  ISBN 1-4051-0402-3 (pbk.)
  1. Communicable diseases in children—Outlines, syllabi, etc.
  2. Communicable diseases in children—Handbooks, manuals, etc.
    [DNLM: 1. Communicable Diseases—Child—Handbooks.
2. Communicable Diseases—Child—Outlines. 3. Communicable Diseases—Infant—Handbooks. 4. Communicable Diseases—Infant—Outlines.
5. Pediatrics—methods—Handbooks. 6. Pediatrics—methods—Outlines.
WS 39 B658 2005] I. Title: Pediatric infectious diseases. II. Shah, Samir S.
III. Series.

RJ401.B584 2005
618.22'9–dc22

                                                                    2004013358
A catalogue record for this title is available from the British Library

Acquisitions: Beverly Copland
Development: Selene Steneck
Production: Debra Murphy
Cover design: Hannus Design Associates
Interior design: Mary McKeon
Illustrations: Electronic Illustrators Group
Typesetter: International Typesetting and Composition in Ft. Lauderdale, FL
Printed and bound by Capital City Press in Berlin, VT

For further information on Blackwell Publishing, visit our website:
www.blackwellmedstudent.com

This book is dedicated to my grandparents—
Shantilal and Savitaben Shah and Ramanlal and Savitaben Sheth

Contents

Contributors

Elizabeth R. Alpern, MD, MSCE
Assistant Professor of Pediatrics
University of Pennsylvania School of Medicine
Philadelphia, Pennsylvania
Attending Physician
Division of Emergency Medicine
The Children's Hospital of Philadelphia
Philadelphia, Pennsylvania

Timothy Andrews, MD
Fellow, Allergy and Immunology
The Children's Hospital of Philadelphia
Philadelphia, Pennsylvania

Robert S. Baltimore, MD
Professor of Pediatrics and Epidemiology
Yale University School of Medicine
New Haven, Connecticut
Attending Pediatrician
Yale-New Haven Children's Hospital
New Haven, Connecticut

Louis M. Bell, MD
Professor of Pediatrics
University of Pennsylvania School of Medicine
Philadelphia, Pennsylvania
Chief, Division of General Pediatrics
The Children's Hospital of Pennsylvania
Philadelphia, Pennsylvania

Jeffrey M. Bergelson, MD
Associate Professor of Pediatrics
University of Pennsylvania School of Medicine
Philadelphia, Pennsylvania
Division of Infectious Diseases
The Children's Hospital of Philadelphia
Philadelphia, Pennsylvania

Matthew J. Bizzarro, MD
Fellow-Neonatology
Yale-New Haven Hospital
New Haven, Connecticut

Kurt A. Brown, MD
Associate Director Clinical Research
AstraZeneca LP
Wilmington, Delaware

Susan Coffin, MD, MPH
Assistant Professor, Department of Pediatrics
University of Pennsylvania School of Medicine
Philadelphia, Pennsylvania
Attending Physician
The Children's Hospital of Philadelphia
Philadelphia, Pennsylvania

Reza J. Daugherty, MD
Instructor of Pediatrics
University of Pennsylvania School of Medicine
Philadelphia, Pennsylvania
Fellow, Pediatric Emergency Medicine
The Children's Hospital of Philadelphia
Philadelphia, Pennsylvania

Arlene Dent, MD, PhD
Fellow, Department of Pediatrics
Case Western Reserve University
Cleveland, Ohio
Fellow, Division of Infectious Diseases
Rainbow Babies and Children's Hospital
Cleveland, Ohio

Dennis R. Durbin, MD, MSCE
Associate Professor of Pediatrics and Epidemiology
University of Pennsylvania School of Medicine
Philadelphia, Pennsylvania
Attending Physician, Emergency Department
The Children's Hospital of Philadelphia
Philadelphia, Pennsylvania

Stephen C. Eppes, MD
Clinical Associate Professor of Pediatrics
Jefferson Medical College
Philadelphia, Pennsylvania

Associate Director, Infectious Diseases
Alfred I. DuPont Hospital for Children
Wilmington, Delaware

Patrick G. Gallagher, MD
Associate Professor
Department of Pediatrics
Yale University School of Medicine
New Haven, Connecticut
Attending Physician
Yale-New Haven Hospital
New Haven, Connecticut

Andrew L. Garrett, MD, FAAP, EMT
Instructor in Pediatrics and Emergency Medicine
University of Massachusetts Medical School
Worcester, Massachusetts
Fellow in EMS and Disaster Medicine
Attending Physician in Pediatric Emergency Medicine
University of Massachusetts Memorial Health Care
Worcester, Massachusetts

Laura Gomez, MD
Department of Pediatrics
Thomas Jefferson University
Philadelphia, Pennsylvania
Alfred I. DuPont Hospital for Children
Wilmington, Delaware

Jane M. Gould, MD, FAAP
Attending Physician
The Children's Hospital of Philadelphia
Philadelphia, Pennsylvania

Richard L. Hodinka, PhD
Associate Professor, Pediatrics
University of Pennsylvania School of Medicine
Philadelphia, Pennsylvania
Director, Clinical Virology
The Children's Hospital of Philadelphia
Philadelphia, Pennsylvania

Ron Keren, MD, MPH
Assistant Professor of Pediatrics
University of Pennsylvania School of Medicine
Philadelphia, Pennsylvania

Attending Physician
The Children's Hospital of Philadelphia
Philadelphia, Pennsylvania

Leila M. Khazaeni, MD
Assistant Instructor, Department of Ophthalmology
University of Pennsylvania School of Medicine
Philadelphia, Pennsylvania
Resident
Scheie Eye Institute
Philadelphia, Pennsylvania

Jean O. Kim, MD
Pediatric Infectious Disease Specialist
Germbusters, P.C.
Hoffman Estates, Illinois

Petar Mamula, MD
Assistant Professor of Pediatrics
University of Pennsylvania School of Medicine
Philadelphia, Pennsylvania
Attending Physician, Division of Gastroenterology and Nutrition
The Children's Hospital of Philadelphia
Philadelphia, Pennsylvania

Marian G. Michaels, MD, MPH
Associate Professor of Pediatrics and Surgery
University of Pittsburgh School of Medicine
Pittsburgh, Pennsylvania
Allergy, Immunology and Infectious Diseases
Children's Hospital of Pittsburgh
Pittsburgh, Pennsylvania

Monte D. Mills, MD
Director of Ophthalmology
The Children's Hospital of Philadelphia
Philadelphia, Pennsylvania

Karin L. McGowan, PhD, F(AAM)
Associate Professor
Department of Pediatrics
University of Pennsylvania School of Medicine
Philadelphia, Pennsylvania
Director, Microbiology
The Children's Hospital of Philadelphia
Philadelphia, Pennsylvania

Susmita Pati, MD, MPH
Assistant Professor of Pediatrics
University of Pennsylvania School of Medicine
Philadelphia, Pennsylvania
Attending Physician
The Children's Hospital of Philadelphia
Philadelphia, Pennsylvania

Elena Elizabeth Perez, MD, PhD
Fellow, Allergy and Immunology
The Children's Hospital of Philadelphia
Philadelphia, Pennsylvania

Shruti M. Phadke, MD
Assistant Professor of Pediatrics
University of Pittsburgh School of Medicine
Pittsburgh, Pennsylvania
Attending Physician
The Children's Hospital of Pittsburgh
Pittsburgh, Pennsylvania

Anne F. Reilly, MD, MPH
Assistant Professor of Pediatrics
University of Pennsylvania School of Medicine
Philadelphia, Pennsylvania
Attending Oncologist
The Children's Hospital of Philadelphia
Philadelphia, Pennsylvania

David Rubin, MD, MSCE
Assistant Professor of Pediatrics
University of Pennsylvania School of Medicine
Philadelphia, Pennsylvania
Attending Pediatrician
Division of General Pediatrics
The Children's Hospital of Philadelphia
Philadelphia, Pennsylvania

Richard M. Rutstein, MD
Associate Professor of Pediatrics
University of Pennsylvania School of Medicine
Philadelphia, Pennsylvania
Medical Director, Special Immunology Service
Division of General Pediatrics
The Children's Hospital of Philadelphia
Philadelphia, Pennsylvania

John R. Schreiber, MD, MPH
Ruben Bentson Professor and Head Department of Pediatrics
University of Minnesota School of Medicine
Minneapolis, Minnesota

Deborah Blecker Shelly, MS
Supervisor of Clinical Microbiology
The Children's Hospital of Philadelphia
Philadelphia, Pennsylvania

Raman Sreedharan, MD, MRCPCH
Resident in Pediatrics
The Children's Hospital of Philadelphia
Philadelphia, Pennsylvania

Nicholas Tsarouhas, MD
Associate Professor of Pediatrics
University of Pennsylvania School of Medicine
Philadelphia, Pennsylvania
Attending Physician, Emergency Medicine
The Children's Hospital of Philadelphia
Philadelphia, Pennsylvania

Theoklis E. Zaoutis, MD
Assistant Professor of Pediatrics
University of Pennsylvania School of Medicine
Director of Antimicrobial Stewardship
Attending Physician, Division of Infectious Diseases
The Children's Hospital of Philadelphia
Philadelphia, Pennsylvania

Reviewers

Ricky Choi
Class of 2004
Medical University of South Carolina
Charleston, South Carolina

Innocent Monya-Tambi
Class of 2004
Howard University College of Medicine
Washington, DC

John Nguyen, MD
PGY-I
Internal Medicine Prelim/Ophthalmology
University of Texas Medical Branch
Houston, Texas

Nkiruka Ohameje, MPH
Class of 2004
Drexel University College of Medicine
Philadelphia, Pennsylvania

Christian Ramers, MD
Resident, Medicine-Pediatrics
Duke University Medical Center
Durham, North Carolina

Derek Wayman, MD
Resident, Family Practice
University of North Dakota
Grand Forks, North Dakota

Foreword

The disciplines of infectious diseases is a holdout from times past compared with other subspecialties. Clinical skills are not supplanted by technology and procedures. Honing in on cardinal symptoms and the timeline, cadence and context of illness; judging the child's sense of well being; seeking clues on examination to target organ systems involved; cataloging exanthems and enanthems; confirming the clinical suspicion with a few well-chosen tests; and then almost always having highly effective treatment to offer or predicting self-resolution of the illness—the practice of pediatric infectious diseases is challenging and rewarding every day. It has the structure of a puzzle and the richness of human interaction.

Blueprints *Pediatric Infectious Diseases* gets you started with a framework of organ-based diseases, an approach to clinical and laboratory diagnosis, and a short list of empiric treatments. Its broad scope, consistent format, and succinct entries are a great match for a student's need-to-know. It will be a valuable pocket reference for those taking a clinical rotation in pediatric infectious diseases or seeking a primer in the subspecialty.

Sarah S. Long, MD
Professor of Pediatrics
Drexel University College of Medicine

Chief, Section of Infectious Diseases
Philadelphia, PA

Preface

Blueprints have become the standard for medical students to use during their clerkship rotations and sub-internships and as a review book before taking the USMLE Steps 2 and 3.

Blueprints initially were only available for the five main specialties: medicine, pediatrics, obstetrics and gynecology, surgery, and psychiatry. Students found these books so valuable that they asked for Blueprints in other topics and so family medicine, emergency medicine, neurology, cardiology, and radiology were added.

In an effort to answer a need for high yield review books for the elective rotations, Blackwell Publishing now brings you Blueprints in pocket size. These books are developed to provide students in the shorter, elective rotations, often taken in 4th year, with the same high yield, essential contents of the larger Blueprint books. These new pocket-sized Blueprints will be invaluable for those students who need to know the essentials of a clinical area but were unable to take the rotation. Students in physician assistant, nurse practitioner, and osteopath programs will find these books meet their needs for the clinical specialties.

Feedback from student reviewers gave high praise for this addition to the Blueprints brand. Each of these new books was developed to be read in a short time period and to address the basics needed during a particular clinical rotation. Please see the Series Page for a list of the books that will soon be in your bookstore.

Acknowledgments

The conceptual basis for this book arose from my teaching experiences at The Children's Hospital of Philadelphia. The housestaff and medical students asked insightful questions (occasionally at 3 a.m.) that provided the initial stimulus for this book. I am indebted to them for this inspiration.

I thank my colleagues who have contributed their expertise in writing chapters for this book. I would also like to thank my Department Chair, Dr. Alan Cohen, and my Division Chiefs, Drs. Louis Bell and Paul Offit, for creating an environment supportive of intellectual pursuits. During the years, I have learned from many other excellent clinicians. Their dedication to teaching and commitment to patient care are attributes I strive to emulate. Without them, this accomplishment would not be possible. There is not enough space to list you all by name but know that I consider learning from you a privilege. Marie Egan, Victor Morris, Patrick Gallagher, Stephen Ludwig, Bill Schwartz, and Istvan Seri deserve special recognition for sharing their wisdom and experience as I embark on my career.

Beverly Copland and Selene Steneck, my editors at Blackwell Publishing, demonstrated remarkable enthusiasm and extraordinary patience as this book developed. My thanks also extend to the staff members at Blackwell Publishing who contributed to the production, marketing, and distribution of this book.

My family has provided unwavering support for all of my projects. I cannot find words sufficient to express my appreciation. Finally, I offer my thanks to my friends and colleagues who have supported, counseled, and nurtured me during this time. You have my heartfelt gratitude.

—Samir S. Shah, M.D.

Abbreviations

5-FC	5-fluorocytosine
AAP	American Academy of Pediatrics
Ab	Antibody
ABPA	Allergic bronchopulmonary aspergillosis
AFB	Acid-fast bacillus
Ag	Antigen
ALC	Absolute lymphocyte count
ALT	Elevated alanine aminotransferase
ANC	Absolute neutrophil count
AOM	Acute otitis media
ARDS	Acute respiratory distress syndrome
ART	Antiretroviral therapy
ASD	Atrial septal defect
ASO	Antistreptolysin O
AST	Aspartate-aminotransferase
BAL	Bronchoalveolar lavage
BAT	Botulinum antitoxin
BCYE	Buffered Charcoal Yeast Extract
BDNA	Branched DNA signal amplification
BSA	Body surface area
BW	Biological warfare
cAb	Core antibody
CBC	Complete blood count
CDC	Centers for Disease Control and Prevention
CFTR	Cystic fibrosis transmembrane conductance regulator
CGD	Chronic granulomatous disease
CHD	Congenital heart disease
CIN	Cefsulodin-irgasan-novobiocin
CLD	Chronic lung disease
CMV	Cytomegalovirus
CNS	Central nervous system
CoNS	Coagulase-negative staphylococci
CPE	Cytopathic effect
CRMO	Chronic recurrent multifocal osteomyelitis
CRP	C-reactive protein
CSF	Cerebrospinal fluid
CT	Computed tomography
CVA	Cerebrovascular accident
CVC	Central venous catheter
CVID	Common variable immune deficiency

CXR	Chest radiograph
DCF	Dichlorohydrofluorescein
DDS	Dose dependent susceptible
DFA	Direct fluorescent antibody
DHR	Dihydroxyrhodamine 123
DIC	Disseminated intravascular coagulation
ds	Double stranded
DTP	Diphtheria-tetanus-pertussis (vaccine)
EBV	Epstein-Barr virus
ECG	Electrocardiogram
EEE	Eastern equine encephalitis virus
EEG	Electroencephalogram
EIA	Enzyme immunoassay
ELISA	Enzyme-linked immunosorbent assay
EM	Erythema migrans
EMB	Eosin-methylene blue
ESR	Erythrocyte sedimentation rate
5-FC	5-Fluorocytosine, flucytosine
FISH	Fluorescent in situ hybridization
FMF	Familial Mediterranean fever
FTA-ABS	Fluorescent treponemal antibody absorption test
FUO	Fever of unknown origin
GAS	Group A *Streptococcus*
GBS	Group B *Streptococcus*
GGT	γ-Glutamyltransferase
GI	Gastrointestinal
GMS	Gomori methenamine silver
GNR	Gram-negative rods
GU	Genitourinary
HAV	Hepatitis A virus
Hb SS	Sickle cell disease
BIG-IV	Botulinum immune globulin
HBIG	Hepatitis B immune globulin
HBV	Hepatitis B virus
HCV	Hepatitis C virus
HDCV	Human diploid cell vaccine
HDV	Hepatitis D virus
HEV	Hepatitis E virus
HHV-6	Human herpes virus 6
HHV-7	Human herpesvirus 7
HHV-8	Human herpes virus 8
HIB	*Haemophilus influenzae* type b
HIV	Human immunodeficiency virus
HPV	Human papilloma virus
HSM	Hepatosplenomegaly
HSV	Herpes simplex virus
HTLV	Human T-cell lymphotropic virus
IFA	Indirect fluorescent antibody

Ig	Immunoglobin
IgA	Immunoglobulin A
IgE	Immunoglobulin E
IgG	Immunoglobulin G
IgM	Immunoglobulin M
INH	Isoniazid
IUGR	Intrauterine growth retardation
IVIG	Intravenous immunoglobulin
JCAHO	Joint Commission on Accreditation of Healthcare Organizations
JRA	Juvenile rheumatoid arthritis
KOH	Potassium hydroxide
LCMV	Lymphocytic choriomeningitis virus
LCR	Ligase chain reaction
LDH	Lactate dehydrogenase
LIP	Lymphocytic interstitial pneumonitis
LP	Lumbar puncture
Mac −	No growth on MacConkey agar
Mac +	Growth on MacConkey agar (as opposed to blood agar)
MBC	Minimal bactericidal concentration
MCT	Mother-child transmission
MHA-TP	Microhemagglutination for *Treponema pallidum*
MIC	Minimal inhibitory concentration
MMR	Measles-mumps-rubella (vaccine)
MRI	Magnetic resonance imaging
MRSA	Methicillin-resistant *Staphylococcus aureus*
MSSA	Methicillin-sensitive *Staphylococcus aureus*
N/A	Not applicable (no form of this disease exists)
NASBA	Nucleic acid sequence–based amplification
NBT	Nitroblue tetrazolium
NP	Nasopharyngeal
NSAID	Nonsteroidal anti-inflammatory drug
NTM	Nontuberculous mycobacteria
O&P	Ova and parasite
OB	Occult bacteremia
OI	Opportunistic infections
OM	Otitis media
OME	Otitis media with effusion
PBP	Penicillin-binding proteins
PCN	Penicillin
PCP	*Pneumocystis carinii* pneumonia
PCR	Polymerase chain reaction
PE	Progressive encephalopathy
PEP	Postexposure prophalaxis
PFAPA	Periodic fever, aphthous stomatitis, pharyngitis, and cervical adentitis
PFGE	Pulsed-field electrophoresis

PICC	Peripherally inserted central catheter
PID	Pelvic inflammatory disease
PPD	Purified protein derivative (for tuberculin skin test)
PT	Prothrombin time
PTLD	Posttransplantation lymphoproliferative disorders
PTT	Partial thromboplastin time
RIG	Rabies immune globulin
RMSF	Rocky Mountain spotted fever
RPR	Rapid plasma reagin
RSV	Respiratory syncytial virus
RTI	Reverse transcriptase inhibitor
sAb	Surface antibody
sAg	Surface antigen
SARS	Sudden acute respiratory syndrome
SBE	Subacute bacterial endocarditis
SBI	Serious bacterial infections
SBP	Primary spontaneous bacterial peritonitis
SCID	Severe combined immunodeficiency
SDA	Strand displacement amplification
SE	Southeast
seg	Segmented
SHEA	Society for Healthcare Epidemiology in America
SIRS	Systemic inflammatory response syndrome
SLV	St. Louis encephalitis virus
SPACE	*Serratia, Pseudomonas, Acinetobacter, Citrobacter,* and *Enterobacter species*
SPN	*Streptococcus pneumoniae*
ss	Single stranded
STD	Sexually transmitted disease
TB	Tuberculosis
TIG	Tetanus immune globulin
TMA	Transcription-mediated amplification
TMP-SMX	Trimethoprim-sulfamethoxazole
TNF-α	Tumor necrosis factor-α
TRAPS	Tumor necrosis factor receptor–associated periodic syndrome (formerly Hibernian fever)
TSS	Toxic shock syndrome
TT	Tube thoracostomy
UA	Urinalysis
URI	Upper respiratory infection
UTI	Urinary tract infection
VAERS	Vaccine Adverse Event Reporting System
VATS	Video-assisted thoracoscopy
VCUG	Voiding cystourethrogram
VDRL	Venereal Disease Research Laboratory
VEE	Venezuelan encephalitis
VHF	Viral hemorrhagic fevers
VL	Viral load

VP	Ventriculoperitoneal
VSD	Ventricular septal defect
VUR	Vesicoureteral reflux
VZIG	Varicella-zoster immune globulin
VZV	Varicella-zoster virus
WB	Western blot
WBC	White blood cell count
WEE	Western equine encephalitis virus
WNV	West Nile virus
XLA	X-linked agammaglobulinemia

1 Diagnostic Microbiology

Karin L. McGowan, PhD, F(AAM) and Deborah Blecker Shelly, MS

BACTERIA

Laboratory Methods Used to Identify Bacteria

Microscopy/Direct Examination (Table 1-1)

- Gram stain: Bacteria stain differently based on cell wall composition
  - Gram positive: Stain purple/blue; Gram negative: Stain red/pink
  - Damaged or incomplete cell walls (i.e., *Mycoplasma*, *Ureaplasma*) and those with lipids (e.g., *Mycobacteria*) will not stain; *Nocardia* and some fungi stain unpredictably
- Acid-fast stains
  - Auramine-rhodamine (fluorescent): Used for rapid screening; most sensitive
  - Ziehl-Neelsen and Kinyoun (nonfluorescent): Detection of acid-fast bacteria (*Mycobacteria*)
  - Modified Kinyoun (nonfluorescent): Detection of weakly acid-fast bacteria (i.e., *Nocardia, Rhodococcus, Tsukamurella*)

Culture Media

- Routine culture media
  - Blood agar: Supports growth of most common bacteria except *Haemophilus, Neisseria* spp.; can determine hemolysis on blood agar plate
  - Chocolate agar: *Haemophilus, Neisseria* spp.
  - MacConkey and eosin-methylene blue (EMB) agar: Selective and differential for gastrointestinal organisms (enterics) only. Also differentiates lactose fermenters (*Escherichia coli, Klebsiella, Enterobacter*) from non-lactose fermenters (*Salmonella, Shigella, Pseudomonas*)
- Specialized culture media is needed for the following organisms that do no grow on routine media: *Bordetella* spp., *Legionella* spp., *Escherichia coli* O157:H7, *Campylobacter* spp., and *Yersinia* spp.

■ TABLE 1-1 Correlations of Staining Result with Possible Organisms

Preliminary Staining Result	Possible Organisms
Catalase-positive, gram-positive cocci	Staphylococcus, Micrococcus, Aerococcus
Catalase-negative, gram-positive cocci	Streptococcus, Enterococcus, Abiotrophia, Leuconostoc, Pediococcus, Gemella, Aerococcus, Lactococcus, Globicatella
Nonbranching, catalase-positive, gram-positive bacilli	Bacillus, Listeria, Corynebacterium, Kurthia, Turicella
Nonbranching, catalase-negative, gram-positive bacilli	Erysipelothrix, Lactobacillus, Arcanobacterium, Lactobacillus, Gardnerella
Branching or partially acid-fast gram-positive bacilli	Nocardia, Streptomyces, Rhodococcus, Oerskovia, Tsukamurella, Gordona, Rothia
Gram-negative bacilli and coccobacilli (Mac +, oxidase negative)	Enterobacteriaceae, Acinetobacter, Chryseomonas, Flavimonas, Stenotrophomonas
Gram-negative bacilli and coccobacilli (Mac +, oxidase +)	Pseudomonas, Burkholderia, Ralstonia, Achromobacter group, Ochrobactrum, Chryseobacterium, Alcaligenes, Bordetella (excl. B. pertussis), Comamonas, Vibrio, Aeromonas, Plesiomonas, Chromobacterium
Gram-negative bacilli and coccobacilli (Mac −, oxidase +)	Moraxella, elongated Neisseria, Eikenella corrodens, Pasteurella, Actinobacillus, Kingella, Cardiobacterium, Capnocytophaga
Gram-negative bacilli and coccobacilli (Mac −, oxidase variable)	Haemophilus

- Nonculture tests are usually better for detecting the following organisms: *Brucella, Corynebacterium diphtheriae, Coccidioides immitis, Streptobacillus, Francisella tularensis, Bartonella, Afipia, Helicobacter, Chlamydia, Rickettsia, Ehrlichia, Coxiella, Mycoplasma, Ureaplasma, Treponema, Borrelia*

Direct Specimen Diagnostic Testing
- Direct testing of clinical specimen by detection of antigen, DNA, or antibody (Table 1-2)
- Particularly useful for detection of nonculturable, fastidious, slowly growing organisms
- Considerations: 1) interfering substances such as blood may affect result; 2) may represent nonviable organism

Conventional Bacterial Identification Methods
- Conventional: Phenotypic approach observing macroscopic morphology on culture media (hemolysis, non-lactose fermenter, etc.); microscopic staining characteristics (pairs, chains);

■ TABLE 1-2 Examples of Direct Specimen Diagnostic Testing

Infectious Agent	Comments
Bartonella henselae	IFA; sensitivity 95%, specificity 95%
Bordetella pertussis	PCR (new gold standard), DFA
Chlamydia trachomatis	EIA for antigen; DFA, LCR, PCR; DNA probe
Clostridium difficile	Toxin A and B detection
Clostridium botulinum	Toxin detection (stool)
E. coli 0157	EIA for *Shiga* toxin; peak 2–3 weeks after initial infection
Legionella pneumophila	DFA; Urine antigen test detects *L. pneumophila* serogroup 1 (sensitivity 80%)
Mycoplasma pneumoniae	PCR
Neisseria gonorrhoeae	LCR; DNA probe
Streptococcus pneumoniae	Antigen testing (urine); tests positive in vaccinated children
Streptococcus pyogenes	Rapid *Streptococcus* antigen, DNA hybridization, agglutination (ASO)

atmospheric requirements (aerobic, anaerobic, CO_2); plus use of spot tests: oxidase, catalase, indole, etc.

- Commercial systems: Rapid (4 hour) or overnight; automated or nonautomated; substrate utilization, enzyme production, carbohydrate fermentation; biochemical reactions converted to a code compared with large database
- Other: Latex agglutination tests (*Staphylococcus aureus, Campylobacter jejuni, Salmonella/Shigella*), serotyping of *Haemophilus influenzae* (types a, b, c, d, e, f); *Neisseria meningitidis* (Groups A, B, C, X, Y, Z, W135); *Salmonella* and *Shigella* for outbreaks and vaccine efficacy; gas-liquid chromatography, long-chain fatty acid analysis, ribotyping or pulsed-field gel electrophoresis comparing nucleic acids

Identification Methods for Mycobacteria

- Culture on Lowenstein-Jensen media: Examine growth characteristics (rate, pigment production) plus biochemical testing
- Typical growth rates: *M. tuberculosis*: 3 to 4 weeks; *M. avium-intracellulare* complex: 2 weeks; rapidly growing nontuberculous mycobacteria (e.g., *M. abscessus, M. fortuitum, M. chelonae, M. smegmatis*): ≤7 days
- Nucleic acid probes for culture confirmation: Generally for *M. tuberculosis* and *M. avium* complex (*M. avium, M. intracellulare*)
- DNA sequencing: Generally used for other species (i.e., *M. kansasii, M. gordonae*)

Antimicrobial Susceptibility Testing

Specific Susceptibility Tests
- Disc diffusion (Kirby-Bauer): Commercially prepared filter paper disks impregnated with a specified concentration of an antimicrobial agent are applied to the surface of an agar medium inoculated with organism. Drug diffuses into agar and creates a gradient; no growth indicates inhibition
  - Results reported as *Susceptible*, *Intermediate*, or *Resistant*
  - Bacteria are considered susceptible to an antibiotic if *in vitro* growth is inhibited at a concentration one fourth to one eighth that *achievable in the patient's blood*, given a *usual dose* of the antibiotic
- Broth/agar microdilution: Antibiotics at varying concentrations (representing therapeutically achievable ranges) are tested against each organism to determine the minimal inhibitory concentration (MIC), the lowest dilution that inhibits growth
- Gradient diffusion (E Test): Plastic test strip impregnated with a continuous exponential gradient of antibiotic is placed on a Mueller-Hinton plate inoculated with a standard concentration of bacteria; following incubation, a tear-drop–shaped zone of inhibition is observed; point of zone edge intersecting the strip is the MIC
  - Good for fastidious and anaerobic bacteria (i.e., *Streptococcus pneumoniae*)

Other Tests
- Minimal bactericidal concentration (MBC): Defined as the lowest dilution that kills (rather than inhibits the growth of) 99.9% of organisms present
  - MBC is used to detect "tolerance"; defined as MIC/MBC ratio ≥1:32
  - Clinical importance: Tolerance may make "cidal" antibiotics act in a static manner
- Serum cidal test (Schlicter test): Tests the bactericidal activity of patient's serum against a particular organism
  - Clinical importance: Useful with nonfastidious organisms (i.e., *S. aureus*) when issues arise regarding sites with difficult drug penetration (e.g., oral therapy for osteomyelitis)

Blood Cultures

Guidelines
- Greater volume of blood inoculated yields higher sensitivity and faster detection

- Taking multiple specimens increases sensitivity (91.5% detected with first, 99.3% with second, 99.6% by one of first three); draw from two separate sites; time interval not critical
- In pediatrics, anaerobes account for less than 1% of bacteremia; use pediatric rather than separate anaerobic culture bottle
- False-positive (contaminated) blood cultures account for up to 50% of all positive blood cultures; allow povidone-iodine (Betadine) to dry completely
- Detection of subacute bacterial endocarditis (SBE) requires larger volumes of blood; when SBE suspected, obtain three to five blood cultures from different sites within a 24-hour period; 3–5 mL of blood per culture. Agents that cause SBE may require longer incubation times

Methods

- Automated and continuously monitored: These systems automatically detect growth and then generate an alert signal to inform the user that a bottle is positive
  - For example, in the BacT/Alert a sensor located in bottom of the bottle changes color when it detects CO_2 produced by microorganisms. The bottles are scanned every 10 minutes for color change compared with baseline
  - In contrast, the ESP System detects pressure changes in the headspace of blood culture bottle, which indicates microbial gas production or consumption
- Conventional broth bottles (nonautomated): Incubated blood culture bottles are monitored visually daily (not "continuously"). This is a very labor-intensive process but is useful for places with a relatively small number of cultures
- If a lab uses a manual rather than a continuously monitored system, ask when the plates were last examined for growth before determining whether to discontinue antibiotics for "negative" cultures

FUNGI

Classification of Fungi

- Yeasts: Single celled, round, or oval; reproduce by budding
- Molds: Multicellular, composed of tubular structures (hyphae) that grow by branching, produce spores, some are dimorphic (can grow as yeast or mold forms)

Cutaneous/Superficial

- *Candida* spp.: Cutaneous, mucocutaneous, and nail infections; normal skin flora

- *Malassezia furfur* (tinea versicolor): Normal skin flora in fat-rich areas; causes pityriasis versicolor and seborrheic dermatitis when density becomes too high
- *Exophiala werneckii* (tinea nigra): Black rings on skin
- Dermatophytes ("ringworm"): Skin/hair/nail infections from molds *Microsporum* spp., *Trichophyton* spp., *Epidermophyton*. Caused by contact with spores via animals or people

Subcutaneous

- Sporotrichosis (*Sporothrix schenkii*): Chronic subcutaneous fungal infection that invades regional lymphatics, caused by traumatic inoculation with rose thorns

Endemic/Systemic Mycoses

Acquired through inhalation or inoculation of spores; all are dimorphic, meaning they exist in more than one physical form (mold, yeast, spherule); most localized to an endemic zone. Most occur as primary pulmonary infections with rare dissemination (central nervous system, skin, bone, lymph nodes, viscera), except in immunocompromised hosts and very young children.

- *Blastomyces dermatitidis:* Southeastern United States as far north as Norfolk, VA; Ohio, Mississippi, Missouri, and Arkansas river valleys
- *Coccidioides immitis:* California, Arizona, New Mexico, Texas, Mexico, South America
- *Histoplasma capsulatum:* Ohio; Missouri; Mississippi river valleys; Lancaster County, PA; New York State; southern Canada; Central and South America
- *Paracoccidioides brasiliensis:* Central and South America
- *Penicillium marneffei:* Cambodia, southern China, Indonesia, Laos, Malaysia, Thailand, and Vietnam
- *Sporothrix schenkii:* Worldwide

Opportunistic Fungi

In theory, any yeast or mold can cause systemic disease in a compromised host; the most commonly seen yeasts and molds are listed here.

- *Candida* spp.: *C. albicans* and *C. parapsilosis* most common; cause many types of infections, including dissemination to heart, lung, liver, spleen, and kidney after catheter-related fungemia
- *Aspergillus* spp.: Ubiquitous in environment; cause disease (especially in sinuses and lungs) in cases of prolonged neutropenia, bone marrow and solid organ transplantation, and neutrophil dysfunction (e.g., chronic granulomatous disease)
- Zygomycetes (*Mucor, Absidia, Rhizopus*): Diabetics and immunosuppressed receiving steroids at highest risk

- *Cryptococcus neoformans:* Inhaled from pigeon droppings; causes pneumonia and meningitis in human immunodeficiency virus (HIV) and organ transplantation patients; large dose can infect a normal host
- *Fusarium* spp.: Leukemia and bone marrow transplantation patients at highest risk
- *Malassezia furfur:* Receiving intravenous lipids is a major risk factor, seen mostly in neonates

Laboratory Methods Used to Identify Fungi

Microscopy/Direct Examination
Some commonly used fungal stains discussed below.

- Giemsa: Best for visualization of fungi seen in bone marrow aspirate specimens and blood smears (e.g., *H. capsulatum* and *P. marneffei*)
- Gomori methenamine silver (GMS): Most popular pathology stain for visualizing yeast or hyphae in tissue; excellent for *Pneumocystis carinii*
- Gram stain: Detects *Candida* spp.
- Modified acid-fast bacillus (modified AFB): Performed directly on specimens and on colonies from culture; *Nocardia* spp. are positive, *Actinomyces* and *Streptomyces* are negative
- Potassium hydroxide (KOH) 10%: Most popular stain to demonstrate fungi in hair, skin, and nail specimens

Identification Methods for Fungi
- Molds:
  - *Aspergillus: Septate 45° angle* branching hyphae on histology; Zygomycetes: *nonseptate 90° angle* branching hyphae on histology
  - *Aspergillus*: Characteristic conidiophores (from biopsy specimen) are usually present within 48 hours on Sabouraud dextrose or brain-heart infusion agar. In contrast to candidiasis, blood cultures almost never positive in invasive aspergillosis
  - With some groups of molds and the filamentous bacteria (*Nocardia, Streptomyces, Actinomyces*) biochemical tests identify an isolate; such testing can take from 2 to 10 days
  - Extent to which a mold should be identified (genus vs. genus and species) depends on site of isolation and immune status of the host
- Yeast:
  - Pseudohyphae on Gram stain of surface lesions or aspirated fluids or GMS stain of biopsy specimens suggests *C. albicans*
  - Microscopically, examine yeast for presence of capsule by India ink (*C. neoformans*)

- *Candida* spp. appear as pearly white colonies with a sharply demarcated border on blood or Sabouraud dextrose agar
- CHROMagar Candida differentiates *Candida albicans*, *Candida tropicalis*, and *Candida krusei* by color and morphology in 24 to 48 hours
- *Candida* spp. usually begin to grow within 48 hours in standard blood culture bottles; may grow more quickly under lysis centrifugation (blood mixed with lysing agent is plated directly onto appropriate culture media)
- Yeast identification takes 4 hours to 3 days depending on the system and species

- Endemic/dimorphic fungi:
  - Slow growth rates and (5 days to 8 weeks)
  - A specific exoantigen test and/or DNA probe can be used to identify *Blastomyces*, *Coccidioides*, *Histoplasma*, and *Paracoccidioides*

Antigen, Metabolite (Chemical), and Antibody Detection

- *Aspergillus* spp. and *Candida:* Antigen and metabolite tests have low sensitivity in cases of invasive disease and so are rarely used
- *C. neoformans:* Antigen test commonly used; detects capsular polysaccharide antigen, high sensitivity (99%); usually sent from CSF and blood in conjunction with culture
- *H. capsulatum:* Antigen test commonly used; detects heat-stable polysaccharide in serum, urine, and cerebrospinal fluid (CSF); urine 99% sensitive for disseminated disease but less than 50% sensitive for local pulmonary disease; always confirm with culture since antigen test cross reacts with other dimorphic fungi. *Histoplasma* urinary antigen test best for patients unable to mount sufficient antibody response (e.g., HIV infection)
- Antibody detection commonly used for blastomycosis, coccidioidomycosis, histoplasmosis, and paracoccidioidomycosis.

Antifungal Susceptibility Testing

- Standardized methods now available for quantitative antifungal susceptibility testing of yeast and some molds, but clinical correlation data are lacking

PARASITES

Classification of Parasites

Protozoa

- Single-celled organisms and some have two physical forms: An adult form called a trophozoite and a "resting" form called a cyst. Divided into six classes (Table 1-3)

■ TABLE 1-3 Clinically Encountered Protozoa	
Class	**Common Clinical Examples**
Amebae	*Entamoeba histolytica, Naegleria, Acanthamoeba, Blastocystis hominis*
Ciliates	*Balantidium coli*
Flagellates	*Giardia lamblia, Chilomastix mesnili, Dientamoeba fragilis, Leishmania* spp., *Trypanosoma* spp., *Trichomonas vaginalis*
Coccidia	*Cryptosporidium, Cyclospora, Isospora, Toxoplasma gondii*
Sporozoa	*Plasmodium* spp., *Babesia* spp.
Microsporidia	*Enterocytozoon bieneusi, Encephalitozoon* spp.

- There are many saprophytic protozoa that laboratories report if found in human stool; their presence indicates that a patient has ingested contaminated food or water. These include *Entamoeba coli, E. dispar, E. hartmanni, Endolimax nana*, and *Iodamoeba butschlii*
- *Blastocystis hominis* is considered a saprophyte if present in small numbers; if present in moderate or large numbers, treatment should be implemented

Helminths (worms)
- Nematodes (roundworms): Intestinal and blood forms; separated by how they enter the host:
  - Humans ingest ova: *Enterobius vermicularis* (pinworm), *Trichuris trichiura* (whipworm), *Ascaris lumbricoides* (human roundworm)
  - Humans ingest larvae: *Trichinella, Anisakis*
  - Larvae burrow into skin from soil: Hookworm, *Strongyloides*
  - Humans acquire via insect bite: Microfilaria (*Wuchereria bancrofti, Loa loa, Mansonella* spp.)
  - Animal nematodes that accidentally infect humans: *Ancylostoma brasiliense* (dog and cat hookworm penetrates human skin to cause cutaneous larva migrans) and *Toxocara canis* and *T. cati* (dog and cat roundworms; humans ingest ova to cause visceral or ocular larva migrans)
- Cestodes (tapeworms; flat worms): Come in intestinal and tissue forms
  - Intestinal infection in humans after ingestion of infected fish (*Diphyllobothrium latum*), arthropods (*Hymenolepis nana, Hymenolepis diminuta*), pork (*Taenia solium*), or beef (*T. saginata*)
  - Tissue infection in humans after ingestions of eggs from infected human (*T. solium*) or sheep (*Echinococcus granulosus*) stool

- Trematodes (flukes): come in intestinal, liver, lung, and blood forms
  - Intestinal: *Fasciolopsis buski*, *Echinostoma ilocanum*, *Heterophyes heterophyes*, *Metagonimus yokogawai*; acquired by ingestion of infected raw/undercooked water chestnuts, bamboo shoots, mollusks, or freshwater fish
  - Liver and lung: *Clonorchis sinensis*, *Opisthorchis viverrini*, *Fasciola hepatica* (liver), *Paragonimus* spp. (lung); acquired by ingesting infected raw fish or water plants
  - Blood: *Schistosoma mansoni*, *S. mekongi*, *S. haematobium*, *S. intercalatum*; acquired when the microscopic cercarial form liberated from fresh water snails penetrates human skin

Arthropods (Medically Important)

An enormous group that cannot be thoroughly covered in this text. Medically important arthropods transmit disease to humans either by serving as vectors in another parasite's life cycle or by causing disease directly through their bites (e.g., *Anopheles* mosquito transmits malaria).

Laboratory Methods to Identify Parasites

Morphologic Identification: Ova and Parasite (O&P) Examination

- Most parasites still identified by their macroscopic and microscopic morphology
- O&P consists of three separate parts: Stool is 1) *grossly examined* for worms and worm segments; 2) *concentrated* to maximize finding ova and larvae; and 3) *stained* to maximize finding intestinal protozoa
  - Routine O&P does not include *Cyclospora* and Microsporidia
  - Sputum: Examined microscopically to detect migrating larvae of *A. lumbricoides*, hookworm, and *Strongyloides*; protozoa *E. histolytica*, *Cryptosporidium parvum*, *P. carinii* (now classified as a fungus); eggs of *Paragonimus* and *Echinococcus*
  - Blood, bone marrow: Examined microscopically to detect *Plasmodium* spp., *Babesia* spp., *Trypanosoma* spp., and *Leishmania* spp.
  - Laboratory should be notified at the time the specimen is submitted when *Acanthamoeba* or *Naegleria* are suspected in CSF
  - Polymerase chain reaction used for *Toxoplasma gondii*

Microscopy/Direct Examination

- Giemsa stain: Best stain for all blood parasites and microfilaria, *Acanthamoeba*, *Naegleria*, Microsporidia, *Toxoplasma*, *P. carinii*

- AFB and modified acid-fast stains: *Cryptosporidium, Cyclospora, Isospora,* Microsporidia
- Silver stains: *P. carinii*
- Hematoxylin-based stains: Microfilariae
- Hematoxylin-eosin: *Acanthamoeba, E. histolytica, Trichinella spiralis,* or *Trypanosoma cruzi* in muscle
- Calcofluor white stain: *Naegleria, Acanthamoeba, P. carinii*
- Trichrome or iron hematoxylin: Intestinal tract specimens
- Modified trichrome: Microsporidia
- Fluorescent antibody reagents (direct and indirect): *Giardia lamblia, P. carinii, C. parvum*

Antigen and Antibody Detection

- Antigen and metabolite detection (rapid tests): Designed to detect organisms of high incidence not to replace traditional O&P if you are looking for the unusual
  - Antigen tests commonly used for *C. parvum*; *G. lamblia, E. histolytica,* and *Plasmodium* spp. (result but must be supplemented with smears for percent parasitemia; poor at detecting mixed infections)
- Antibody detection: Requires acute and convalescent specimens
  - Commonly used for diagnosis of *Babesia microti* (in conjunction with Wright-stained blood smears), *Echinococcus granulosus* (hepatic cysts more likely to elicit antibody response that pulmonary cysts), *E. histolytica* (useful for extraintestinal infection; positive in 70% with amebic liver abscess), *Leishmania* spp. (antibodies detected during infection in 95% of immunocompetent patients and 50% of HIV patients), microfilariae (elevated IgG_4 levels indicate active infection), *T. canis, T. gondii, T. spiralis, T. cruzi*

2

Diagnostic Virology

Richard L. Hodinka, PhD

Classification and Properties of Viruses
(Tables 2-1 and 2-2)

■ TABLE 2-1 Properties and Classification of DNA Viruses that Cause Human Disease

Family Name	Virus Size (nm)	Naked or Enveloped	Genome	Common Examples
Adenoviridae	70–90	Naked	ds, linear	Adenoviruses
Hepadnaviridae	42	Enveloped	ds, circular	HBV
Herpesviridae	150–200	Enveloped	ds, linear	HSV-1 and -2, CMV, EBV, VZV, HHV-6, HHV-7, HHV-8
Papovaviridae	45–55	Naked	ds, circular	Papillomaviruses, BK and JC polyomaviruses
Parvoviridae	18–26	Naked	ss, linear	Parvovirus B19
Poxviridae	170–200 × 300–450	Enveloped	ds, linear	Smallpox (variola major), vaccinia virus, molluscum contagiosum virus

Laboratory Methods to Identify Viruses

- A variety of methods are available for diagnosis and monitoring of viral diseases (Table 2-3)
- Selection of assays to perform and choice of specimen(s) to collect for testing depend on the patient population and clinical situation and the intended use of the individual tests

Choosing Tests for Viral Detection

- Conventional tube cultures are slow, expensive, and have limited impact on clinical decision making; advantages include high specificity and detection of multiple viruses at one time

■ TABLE 2-2 Properties and Classification of RNA Viruses that Cause Human Disease

Family Name	Virus Size (nm)	Naked or Enveloped	Genome	Common Examples
Arenaviridae	50–300	Enveloped	ss (−), seg	Lassa fever virus, LCMV
Astroviridae	28	Naked	ss, (+)	Astrovirus
Bunyaviridae	90–120	Enveloped	ss (−), seg	Sin Nombre virus, Hantaan virus, Rift Valley fever virus
Caliciviridae	35–40	Naked	ss (+)	Norovirus, calicivirus
Coronaviridae	80–160	Enveloped	ss (+)	SARS coronavirus, other coronaviruses
Filoviridae	80 × 790	Enveloped	ss (−)	Ebola virus, Marburg virus
Flaviviridae	40–50	Enveloped	ss (+)	WNV, SLE virus, dengue virus, HCV, yellow fever virus
Orthomyxoviridae	90–120	Enveloped	ss (−), seg	Influenza virus types A, B, and C
Paramyxoviridae	150–300	Enveloped	ss (−)	RSV, parainfluenza virus types 1, 2, 3, and 4, measles virus, mumps virus, metapneumovirus, Nipah virus
Picornaviridae	28–30	Naked	ss (+)	Enteroviruses, rhinoviruses, HAV
Reoviridae	60–80	Naked	ds, seg	Rotavirus, Colorado tick fever virus
Retroviridae	80–130	Enveloped	ss (+), 2 copies	HIV-1 and 2, HTLV-I and II
Rhabdoviridae	70–85 × 130–380	Enveloped	ss (−)	Rabies virus
Togaviridae	60–70	Enveloped	ss (+)	Rubella virus, EEE virus, WEE virus, VEE virus

(−) or (+) Polarity of single-stranded RNA.

- Shell vial or multiwell plate cultures decrease time required for detection of viruses in culture; detect only one or a few viruses at a time and are normally less sensitive than conventional culture systems

■ TABLE 2-3 Laboratory Methods to Identify Viruses

Method	Organism Detected	Test Format	Test Sensitivity	Time to Result
Cell Culture Systems				
Conventional tube	Live virus	Inoculation of specimens into culture tubes containing human or animal cell monolayers; growth of virus with observation of viral-induced morphologic changes, called cytopathic effects, within cells	High-moderate	Days–weeks
Shell vial or multiwell plate	Live virus	Specimens inoculated onto cell monolayers by centrifugation; viral antigen detected in monolayer using fluorescein-labeled monoclonal antibodies	Moderate	1–5 d
Immunologic Tests				
Immuno-fluorescence	Viral antigen	Fluorescein-labeled monoclonal antibodies bind to viral antigens within infected cells of a clinical specimen	Moderate	1–3 h
Immunoassay	Viral antigen	Monoclonal antibodies conjugated to enzymes or other visualizing molecules and added detector agents bind to viral antigens within infected cells of a clinical specimen	Moderate	20 min–2 h
Nucleic Acid Hybridization Assays				
Conventional	Viral DNA or RNA	Enzyme- or radioactively labeled nucleic acid probes directly bind to viral nucleic acids within clinical material	Low	24 h–several days
Amplification	Viral DNA or RNA	PCR, TMA, NASBA, SDA, bDNA, hybrid capture assays detect viral nucleic acids using target or signal amplification techniques	High	1–2 d
Electron microscopy	Viral particles	Direct visualization of the size and shape of viruses in negatively stained or thin-sectioned specimens	Moderate-low	30 min

(Continued)

■ TABLE 2-3 (Continued)

Method	Detected	Test Format	Test Sensitivity	Time to Result
Cytology	Viral CPE	Examination of Papanicolaou-, hematoxylin-eosin–, or Wright-Giemsa–stained exfoliated cells for direct detection of viral-induced cellular changes	Low	1–2 h
Histology	Viral CPE, Ag, nucleic acids	Hematoxylin-eosin stain or peroxidase-labeled monoclonal antibodies (immunohistochemistry) or nucleic acid probes (in situ hybridization) for direct detection of specific viruses within tissue sections	Moderate-low	1–2 d
Serology	Viral Ab	Mainly immunofluorescence, enzyme immunoassays, and latex agglutination to detect virus-specific IgG or IgM antibody responses	Moderate-low	1–3 h
Genotypic and phenotypic assays	Viral mutations or genetic variants	Sequencing-based molecular tests identify specific gene mutations leading to drug resistance or detect genetic variants that may or may not respond to therapy; culture-based phenotypic assays measure viral replication and resistance in the presence of antiretroviral drugs	High	Genotypic 1–2 d; Phenotypic 2–6 wk

- Use and relative importance of cell culture systems for viral isolation is declining with the continued development of rapid and accurate immunologic and molecular tests
- Immunologic tests for direct detection of viral antigens in clinical material are now commercially available for many viruses, and the assays are routinely used in most clinical laboratories. The tests are rapid, inexpensive, simple to perform, and do not require viable virus for detection; disadvantage of usually being less sensitive than viral culture or molecular amplification techniques
- Conventional nucleic acid hybridization assays have limited utility. Tests are slow, relatively insensitive, cumbersome to perform, and expensive. However, assay format is well suited for detecting human papillomaviruses

- Molecular amplification methods (e.g., PCR) are extremely sensitive and are now the tests of choice for detecting many viruses; quantitative measures of viral nucleic acids (e.g., for CMV, EBV, BK, HCV, HBV, HIV) provide useful information about disease progression, prognosis, transmission, therapeutic response, and development of drug resistance in chronically infected immunocompromised hosts
- Electron microscopy offers the main advantage of speed when doing negative staining of liquid samples (i.e., examining stools for viral agents of gastroenteritis); major limitations include the high cost of the instrument, the requirement for specialized expertise, and the overall lack of sensitivity and specificity. This procedure is seldom available in clinical virology laboratories in the United States
- Direct cytologic or histologic examination of stained clinical material is one of the fastest and oldest methods for detecting viruses. The tests are relatively insensitive in comparison with direct antigen or nucleic acid detection methods. Specificity is also low; for example, Tzanck preparations are limited by their ineffectiveness in distinguishing herpes simplex virus from varicella-zoster virus infections. The sensitivity of histologic staining can be increased somewhat by using immunohisto-chemical or in situ hybridization techniques
- Serological assays provide an indirect diagnostic approach by detecting viral-specific antibody responses. Detection of virus-specific IgM or a seroconversion from a negative to a positive IgG antibody response can be diagnostic of primary infection. Detection of virus-specific IgG in a single serum specimen indicates past exposure or vaccination. Negative antibody titers may exclude viral infection.

Specimen Collecting and Handling for Viral Diagnosis

- Collect specimens as close to clinical onset as possible. Acute viral infections are self-limited and cleared within the first 5 to 10 days of illness. Therefore, nothing is gained by a delay in taking a specimen. However, duration of viral shedding varies depending on the virus, the host immune status, the anatomic site or source of the specimen, and whether there is systemic or local involvement
- Virus recovery may be enhanced by collecting multiple specimens from different body sites
- Transport specimens to the laboratory as quickly as possible after collection because some viruses, particularly those with

envelopes, are quite labile outside their natural host. When immediate transport is not possible, specimens should be kept refrigerated or on wet ice. If delays of 24 to 48 hours are anticipated, rapidly freeze the specimen to –70°C and transport to the laboratory on dry ice. In general, specimens for viral diagnosis should never be stored at room temperature or frozen at –20°C

- Swabs are used for collecting specimens from dermal, rectal, respiratory, and ocular sites. Plastic- or metal-shafted swabs with rayon, Dacron, cotton, or polyester tips should be used; calcium alginate or wood-shafted swabs are inhibitory to some viruses.

- All swab and tissue specimens should be placed in viral transport medium immediately after collection.

- Urine, stool, cerebrospinal fluid, and other body fluid specimens should be submitted to the laboratory in sterile, leak-proof containers. Do not dilute these specimens in viral transport medium.

- Whole blood specimens should be collected in a suitable anticoagulant such as EDTA, sodium heparin, sodium citrate, or acid citrate dextrose. EDTA is currently the preferred anticoagulant for most viral studies that require plasma or white blood cells for testing.

- Specimens for nucleic acid testing (i.e., PCR) should be collected and transported in such a manner as to ensure the stability and amplification of the nucleic acids. This is particularly true when collecting and transporting specimens to detect RNA viruses; RNA is a very unstable molecule and is extremely susceptible to degradation by RNases that are ubiquitous in the environment.

- For serological assays, blood should be collected without the use of anticoagulants or preservatives. A single serum specimen is required to determine the immune status of an individual or for the detection of virus-specific IgM antibody. With few exceptions, paired serum specimens, collected 10–14 days apart, are required for the diagnosis of current or recent viral infections when specimens are tested for virus-specific IgG antibody.

- When submitting specimens to the laboratory, the specimen container should be labeled with the patient's full name, the medical record number or other unique identifier, and date and time of collection. Each specimen should be accompanied by a requisition slip containing the same information as on the specimen as well as the suspected clinical diagnosis.

Antimicrobial Agents

Samir S. Shah, MD

■ BOX 3-1 Ten Questions to Ask Before Prescribing an Antibiotic

1. **How old is the patient?**
   - Pathogens are predictable by age. Also, certain antibiotics are not appropriate for certain age groups (e.g., prolonged doxycycline therapy in a neonate).

2. **What is the site of infection or clinical syndrome?**
   - Pathogens are predictable by site and clinical syndrome.

3. **Does the child have normal or impaired immune defenses (e.g., surgery, immunodeficiency, central venous catheter)?**
   - This may change the likelihood of certain pathogens being present.

4. **Which clinical specimens should be obtained to guide therapy?**
   - Some children require several specimens (e.g., febrile neonate), whereas others require none (e.g., toddler with otitis media).

5. **Which antibiotics have predictable activity against the pathogens considered?**
   - Antibiotics with a relatively narrow spectrum are appropriate in some situations (e.g., a child with streptococcal pharyngitis receives penicillin) but not others (e.g., an infant with suspected meningitis empirically receives vancomycin plus cefotaxime).

6. **Are there local patterns of resistance that I should take into account?**
   - The prevalence of antibiotic-resistant bacteria varies by region.

7. **What special pharmacokinetic/pharmacodynamic properties of an antibiotic are important in regard to this infected site/host?**
   - Some antibiotics do not achieve sufficiently high concentrations at the site of infection (e.g., second-generation cephalosporins are not used to manage meningitis). With some antibiotics adjustment for renal impairment is required (e.g., aminoglycosides).

8. **Is there a drug allergy or drug interaction?**
   - Always ask about medication allergies and know what other medications the patient receives.

9. **Which route of administration would be appropriate for this infection/host?**
   - Consider topical or systemic and intravenous, intramuscular, or oral. The degree of anticipated compliance and ability to absorb certain formulations may factor into this decision (e.g., a child with profuse diarrhea may not absorb sufficient amounts of an orally administered antibiotic).

10. **What is the anticipated duration of therapy?**
    - Always have a planned end point, realizing that it may change depending on the patient's response and many other factors. Issues to consider include the intrinsic pathogenicity of the organism, site of infection, penetration of the antibiotic, use of synergistic combination therapy, and presence of a foreign body.

Mechanisms of Antibiotic Action

Inhibitors of Cell Wall Synthesis
- Mechanism of action: Bind to enzymes involved in cell wall synthesis
    - Natural penicillins
    - Aminopenicillins
    - Antistaphylococcal penicillins
    - Extended spectrum penicillins
    - Cephalosporins (first through fourth generation)
    - Carbapenems
    - Monobactams
    - Vancomycin

Inhibitors of Protein Synthesis
- Mechanism of action: Bind to bacterial ribosomal subunit
    - Aminoglycosides
    - Tetracyclines
    - Macrolides
    - Ketolides
    - Clindamycin
    - Chloramphenicol
    - Oxazolidinones
    - Streptogramins

Inhibitors of Nucleic Acid Synthesis
- Mechanism of action: Interfere with bacterial RNA or DNA synthesis
    - Rifampin
    - Fluoroquinolones

Antimetabolites
- Mechanism of action: Compete with cellular metabolites for attachment to enzyme
    - Trimethoprim-sulfamethoxazole
    - Nitrofurantoin

Mechanisms of Antibiotic Resistance

Bacteria have three main mechanisms of resistance to antibiotics:
1. Alter the antibiotic
2. Alter the antibiotic target site
3. Alter antibiotic transport into or out of the cell
- **Example 1:** Some bacteria produce β-lactamase, a class of enzymes that inactivate β-lactam antibiotics by splitting the β-lactam ring. β-Lactamase: Helps assemble peptidoglycan
    - **Solution:** Couple β-lactamase inhibitors to the β-lactams. Examples include amoxicillin-clavulanate, ampicillin-sulbactam, and piperacillin-tazobactam
- **Example 2:** Penicillin resistance to *Streptococcus pneumoniae* results from alterations in cell wall proteins called penicillin-binding proteins (PBPs). PBP: Cross-links peptidoglycan fragments; number of changes in PBPs determines the level of resistance

- **Solution:** Compensate for inefficient drug binding by increasing amount of drug available. Best example is use of high-dose amoxicillin for otitis media in children at risk for penicillin-resistant *S. pneumoniae* (45 mg/kg/d vs. 90 mg/kg/d). Other example, *S. pneumoniae* resistance to macrolides caused by alteration in one of 30 *erm* (erythromycin ribosome methylation) genes, leading to impaired macrolide binding

- **Example 3:** Mutation in *mef* (membrane efflux) gene causes active macrolide efflux from the cell
  - **Solution:** No great solution. Sometimes an increase in antibiotic concentration alone is not enough to overcome this alteration in antibiotic transport. Occasionally, a specific combination of drugs provides a synergistic antibacterial effect. Other example, carbapenems penetrate OprD porins of many gram-negative rods. Carbapenem-resistant *Pseudomonas aeruginosa* mutants lack OprD

Spectrum of Antibiotic Activity (Table 3-1)

■ TABLE 3-1 Spectrum of Antibiotic Activity

	Penicillin	Ampicillin	Ampicillin-Sulbactam	Oxacillin	Cefazolin (1st)	Cefuroxime (2nd)	Cefotaxime (3rd)	Ceftazidime (3rd)	Cefepime (4th)	Vancomycin	Macrolides
GAS/GBS	++	++	++	++	++	++[1]	++	++	++	++	+
SPN	+	++	++	+	+	+	++	+	++	++	+
Enterococcus	+	++	++	−	−	−	−	−	−	++	−
S. aureus	−	−	++	++	++	++	++	−	++	++	+
MRSA	−	−	−	−	−	−	−	−	−	++	+
Moraxella/ H. influenzae	−	+	++	−	+	++	++	++	++	−	+
E. coli	−	−[2]	+	−	+[3]	+	++	++	++	−	−
K. pneumoniae	−	−	++	−	+	+	++	++	++	−	−
SPACE	−	−	−	−	−	−	+[4]	++	++	−	−
Salmonella	−	+	+	−	+	+	++	++	++	−	−
Anaerobes (mouth)	++	+	++	−	−	−	−	−	−	−	−
Anaerobes (gut)	−	−	++	−	−	−	−	−	−	−	−

(Continued)

TABLE 3-1 (Continued)

	Clinda-mycin	Bactrim	Tetra-cyclines	Metro-nidazole	Amino-glycosides	TICAR-CLAV and PIPTAZO[5]	Carba-penems	Aztreonam	Quinolones	Oxazoli-dinone (Linezolid)	Strepto gramin (Q-D)
GAS/GBS	++	−	−	−	−	++	++	−	+	++	++
SPN	++	−	−[6]	−	−	++	++	−	++	++	++
Enterococcus	−	−[6]	−[6]	−	−[7]	+[8]	++	−	−[6]	++	+
S. aureus	++	+	+	−	−[7]	++	++	−	++	++	++
MRSA	+	++	+	−	−	−	−	−	−	++	++
Moraxella/ H. influenzae	−	++	++	−	++	++	++	++	++	−	+
E. coli/K. pneumoniae	−	+	+	−	++	++	++	++	++	−	−
SPACE	−	+	−	−	++	++	++	++	++	−	−
Salmonella	−	+	−	−	+	+	++	++	++[9]	−	+
Anaerobes (mouth)	++	−	++	++	−	++	++	−	+[9]	++	+
Anaerobes (gut)	++	−	+	++	−	++	++	−	+[9]	−	+

− No or very poor activity against the organism; + May use if sensitivity testing permits; ++ Potential first-line agent

[1] First- and second-generation cephalosporins have very poor CNS penetration. [2] 15% to 50% of E. coli sensitive to ampicillin// [3] 30% to 60% of E. coli and Klebsiella species sensitive to 1st generation cephalosporins// [4] Poor activity vs. P. aeruginosa// [5] Ticarcillin-clavulanate and piperacillin-tazobactam // [6] OK to use for urinary tract infections (except for P. aeruginosa)// [7] OK for synergy but not as monotherapy// [8] Piperacillin-tazobactam more effective than ticarcillin-clavulanate vs. enterococci// [9] Cipro has no anaerobic activity; Levofloxacin covers mouth anaerobes; newer generation quinolones cover both mouth and gut anaerobes.

Antifungal Agents

Theoklis E. Zaoutis, MD

Mechanisms of Antifungal Action and Resistance

- Major differences in the structure of fungi and mammalian cells are relevant to the development and use of antifungal agents
  - Structure: 1) Eukaryotic cell with a nucleus surrounded by nuclear membrane; 2) rigid cell wall composed of chitin, cellulose, or both; 3) cytoplasmic membranes contain sterols

Polyenes
- **Mechanism of action:** Binds to the sterol ergosterol in the fungal cell membrane and causes changes in cell permeability leading to cell lysis and death
- **Mechanism of resistance:** Intrinsic (primary) or acquired (secondary) resistance. Intrinsic observed prior to drug exposure while acquired develops upon exposure to the antifungal agent. Resistance is most commonly associated with altered membrane lipids, particularly ergosterol. Another possible mechanism of resistance is mediated by increased catalase activity
- **Available agents:** Nystatin; amphotericin B; lipid formulations of amphotericin B (amphotericin B lipid complex, amphotericin B cholesteryl sulfate, liposomal amphotericin B)

Azoles
- **Mechanism of action:** Inhibits cytochrome P-450 enzymes used in the synthesis of the fungal cell membrane
- **Mechanism of resistance:** Resistance to azoles can develop by several different mechanisms, including decreased membrane permeability, altered membrane sterols, active efflux, altered or overproduced target enzyme, and compensatory mutations in the desaturase enzyme. The category of DDS (dose dependent susceptible) has been created for azoles to characterize isolates with intermediate resistance that can be inhibited by higher doses of drug. DDS isolates may be treated successfully with 12 mg/kg/d of fluconazole

- **Available agents:** Imidazoles (topical only; ketoconazole, miconazole, clotrimazole); triazoles (fluconazole, itraconazole, voriconazole, posaconazole,* ravuconazole*)

Flucytosine

- **Mechanism of action:** Inhibits RNA and DNA synthesis
- **Mechanism of resistance:** Mechanisms of resistance to flucytosine (5-fluorocytosine, 5-FC) can also be intrinsic or acquired. Intrinsic resistance is seen in *Candida glabrata*. Resistance may be due to the deficiency or lack of enzymes implicated in the metabolism of 5-FC or may be due to deregulation of the pyrimidine biosynthetic pathway. Rapid development of resistance limits the usefulness of 5-FC as a single agent and it should be used in combination with other antifungal agents
- **Available agents:** 5-fluorocytosine (5-FC)

Echinocandins

- **Mechanism of action:** Cyclic lipopeptide structure that inhibits 1,3-β-D-glucan synthase. Glucan is the major component of the fungal cell wall
- **Mechanism of resistance:** Mechanisms of resistance to echinocandins have not been well defined
- **Available agents:** Caspofungin; micafungin*

Allylamines

- **Mechanism of action:** Inhibits squalene epoxidase, an enzyme in the synthetic pathway of the fungal cell membrane
- **Available agents:** Terbinafine; naftifine

Griseofulvin

- **Mechanism of action:** Unknown. The drug is deposited in keratin precursor cells and becomes bound to newly formed keratin, thereby preventing invasion by fungi
- **Available agents:** Griseofulvin (derived from *Penicillium*)

Spectrum of Antifungal Activity

- Spectrum of activity for various antifungal agents is shown in Tables 4-1, 4-2, and 4-3
- Specific recommendations depend on site of infection and host immune status
- Amphotericin B denotes the use of conventional amphotericin B or lipid formulations of amphotericin. At the present time, all formulations of amphotericin are considered therapeutic equivalents

*FDA approval pending.

■ TABLE 4-1 Spectrum of Antifungal Activity Against Yeasts

Yeasts	Amphotericin B	Fluconazole	Voriconazole	Caspofungin	Itraconazole	5-FC*
Candida albicans	S	S	S	S	S	S
C. tropicalis	S	S	S	S	S	S
C. parapsilosis	S	S	S	S	S	S
C. glabrata	S-I	DDS-R	S	S	DDS-R	I-R
C. krusei	S-I	R	S	S	DDS-R	S
C. lusitaniae	R	S	S	R	S	S
Cryptococcus neoformans	S	S	S		S	S

*5-FC should not be used as monotherapy because of the rapid development of resistance.

S, susceptible; I, intermediate; DDS, dose dependent susceptible; R, resistant.

■ TABLE 4-2 Spectrum of Antifungal Activity Against Dimorphic Fungi

Mycosis	Drug of Choice	Alternative
Histoplasma capsulatum	Amphotericin B, itraconazole	Fluconazole
Coccidioides immitis	Amphotericin B, itraconazole, fluconazole, ketoconazole	—
Blastomyces dermatitidis	Amphotericin B, itraconazole	Fluconazole, ketoconazole
Sporothrix schenckii	Amphotericin B, itraconazole	Fluconazole

■ TABLE 4-3 Spectrum of Antifungal Activity Against Molds

Mycosis	Drug of Choice	Alternative
Aspergillus spp.	Voriconazole or amphotericin B	Caspofungin[a]
Fusarium or *Alternaria*[b]	Amphotericin B	Voriconazole
Zygomycetes (Mucorales)	Amphotericin B	None
Malassezia furfur	Fluconazole	Itraconazole

[a] Caspofungin indicated for invasive aspergillosis in patients whose infection is refractory to, or who are intolerant of, other therapies. For dosing guidelines, check with infectious diseases specialists.
[b] Resistant to 5-FC, ketoconazole, fluconazole, echinocandins, miconazole, and itraconazole.

5

Antiviral Agents

Susan Coffin, MD, MPH

Mechanisms of Action of Antiviral Agents

Inhibition of Virus Attachment and Penetration
- Neuraminidase inhibitors
- Interferons

Inhibition of Viral Transcription
- Acyclovir
- Amantidine
- Foscarnet
- Ganciclovir
- Interferons
- Rimantidine
- Nucleoside analogues
- Nucleoside reverse transcriptase inhibitors
- Nonnucleoside reverse transcriptase inhibitors
- Penciclovir
- Ribavirin
- Valacyclovir

Inhibition of Viral Protein Translation and Virion Assembly
- Interferons
- Protease inhibitors

Mechanisms of Resistance to Antiviral Agents

Our understanding of the incidence and mechanisms of antiviral resistance remains incomplete. To date, three main mechanisms of resistance have been identified:

1. Alteration of target site
2. Blocking of drug-induced changes in virus metabolism
3. Inhibition of drug activation

- **Example 1:** HIV-1 develops resistance to nucleoside reverse transcriptase inhibitors by modifying the HIV-1 *pol* gene, which encodes viral reverse transcriptase
  - **Solution:** Combination antiviral therapy will reduce the incidence and rate of HIV resistance to nucleoside reverse transcriptase inhibitors
- **Example 2:** Influenza A resistance to amantidine occurs when mutations in the *M* gene prevent amantidine-induced blockade ion channel function necessary for uncoating of viral genome

TABLE 5-1 Spectrum of Activity for Antiviral Agents for Viral Infections Other Than HIV

	Adenovirus	CMV	EBV	Enterovirus	HBV	HCV	HHV-6	HSV	Influenza A	Influenza B	Parainfluenza	RSV	VZV
Acyclovir	–	–	+	–	–	–	–	++	–	–	–	–	++
Amantadine	–	–	–	–	–	–	–	–	++	–	–	–	–
Cidofovir	+	+	+	–	–	–	–	+	–	–	–	–	+
Famciclovir	–	–	+	–	+	–	+	++	–	–	–	–	–
Foscarnet	–	++	+	–	+	–	+	++	+	+	–	–	+
Ganciclovir	+	++	++	–	–	–	+	+	–	–	–	–	+
Lamivudine	–	–	–	–	++	–	–	–	–	–	–	–	–
Oseltamivir	–	–	–	–	–	–	–	–	++	++	–	–	–
Penciclovir	–	–	–	–	+	–	–	++	–	–	–	–	+
Pleconaril	–	–	–	+	–	–	–	–	–	–	+	–	–
Ribavirin	+	–	–	–	–	+	–	–	+	+	–	++b	–
Rimantadine	–	–	–	–	–	–	–	–	++	–	–	–	–
Valacyclovir	–	–	–	–	–	–	–	++	–	–	–	–	+a
Zanamivir	–	–	–	–	–	–	–	–	++	++	–	–	–

– Not tested or no known activity; + susceptible based on in vitro testing; ++ commonly used for therapy.

a Approved for mangement of herpes zoster.

b Active against RSV, but rarely used because of expense, toxicity, and generally self-limited nature of RSV.

- **Significance:** Almost all influenza viruses isolated from patients who have not received antiviral agents remain susceptible; however, resistant subpopulations of influenza virus may be recovered within 48 hours of treatment with amantidine. The clinical significance of antiviral resistance among influenza viruses remains unclear, although failure of prophylaxis has been reported during several nursing home outbreaks of influenza

- **Example 3:** Mutations in viral thymidine kinase induce herpes simplex virus resistance to acyclovir by inhibiting drug phosphorylation
  - **Solution:** Subtherapeutic concentrations of acyclovir promote the emergence of TK-deficient viruses. Therefore, the use of appropriate drug dosages may reduce the risk of viral resistance

Spectrum of Activity for Antiviral Agents for Viral Infections Other than HIV

The relationship between in vitro susceptibility and clinical response to therapy remains unclear for many antiviral agents (Table 5-1)

6 Ophthalmologic Infections

Leila M. Khazaeni, MD, and Monte D. Mills, MD

Ophthalmia Neonatorum

- Conjunctivitis occurring during the first month of life

■ Epidemiology

- Most common infection occurring during first month of life
- Incidence decreases to less than 1% with ocular prophylaxis (1% tetracycline, 0.5% erythromycin, or 1% silver nitrate)

■ Risk Factors

- Inadequate prenatal screening of the mother for genital infections, failure to receive neonatal ocular prophylaxis
- *Pseudomonas aeruginosa* affects hospitalized premature infants

■ Etiology

- *Chlamydia trachomatis* (8.2/1000 live births) most common in industrialized nations
- Etiologic agents and age of onset: Silver nitrate chemical conjunctivitis (1 day); *Neisseria gonorrhoeae* (3 to 5 days); *C. trachomatis* (5 to 14 days); herpes simplex virus (HSV) (5 to 30 days); bacteria (5 to 14 days; *Staphylococcus aureus*, *Streptococcus pneumoniae*, viridans group streptococci, *Haemophilus influenzae*, *Escherichia coli*, *P. aeruginosa*)

■ Pathogenesis

- Three mechanisms of infection
  - Retrograde spread of organisms to fetal conjunctiva/cornea after premature membrane rupture
  - Direct contact with infected genital secretions during vaginal delivery
  - Direct contact with infected caregivers after birth

■ History/Physical Examination

- Red eye, purulent discharge
- Conjunctival erythema, chemosis, lid edema
- Vesicular eyelid rash with herpes simplex virus (HSV)

■ TABLE 6-1 Testing to Detect Specific Causes of Ophthalmia Neonatorum

Etiologic Agent	Studies	Comments
Chemical	Gram stain	Many neutrophils; must evaluate for other causes
Neisseria gonorrhoeae	Gram stain/culture[a]	Culture on Thayer-Martin medium or chocolate agar
Chlamydia trachomatis[b]	Giemsa stain	Intracytoplasmic inclusion in conjunctival epithelial cells
	Direct fluorescent antibody[a]	Fluorescein-conjugated antibodies stain *Chlamydia* elementary bodies. Also available: enzyme immunoassay and cell culture
Herpes simplex virus	Giemsa stain	Multinucleated giant cells, intranuclear inclusions
	HSV culture[a]	Culture positive within 24–48 h. Also available: direct fluorescent antibody and polymerase chain reaction
Bacteria	Gram stain/culture[a]	Gram stain suggestive; culture confirms etiologic factor(s)

[a] Preferred test.
[b] Specimen must contain conjunctival cells, not exudate alone.

■ Additional Studies (Table 6-1)

■ Differential Diagnosis

• Birth trauma, corneal abrasion, foreign body, nasolacrimal duct obstruction, dacryocystitis, congenital glaucoma

■ Management (Table 6-2)

• In cases of chlamydial or gonococcal conjunctivitis, the mother and her sexual partner require evaluation and treatment for sexually transmitted diseases

■ Complications

• Chemical: None
• *N. gonorrhoeae*: Corneal ulceration or perforation, endophthalmitis, arthritis, sepsis, meningitis
• *C. trachomatis*: Corneal scarring, otitis media, pneumonia. Pneumonia presents at 4 to 12 weeks of life. Findings include staccato cough, tachypnea, and rales without fever

■ **TABLE 6-2 Treatment for Ophthalmia Neonatorum**

Etiologic Agent	Systemic Treatment	Topical Treatment
Chemical	None	None
N. gonorrhoeae	Ceftriaxone × 1 dose Alternative: IV cefotaxime × 7 days	Hourly saline lavage until no further discharge
C. trachomatis	Erythromycin PO × 2–3 weeks	Erythromycin or sulfa ophthalmic ointment

Herpes simplex virus[a]	Acyclovir × 10 days	- Trifluorothymidine
		  1% q 2 h × 7 days
		- Alternative: Vidarabine 3%
		  ointment 5/day × 7 days

Bacteria	None	- Erythromycin or gentamicin ointment

[a] Duration of therapy longer for associated central nervous system or disseminated infection.

- *P. aeruginosa*: Corneal ulceration or perforation; sepsis or meningitis in 40% of premature infants with *P. aeruginosa* conjunctivitis
- HSV: Chorioretinitis, cataracts, corneal scarring

Conjunctivitis in the Older Child

- Inflammation or infection of the conjunctiva.

■ Epidemiology

- Bacterial conjunctivitis usually associated with an upper respiratory infection
- Adenoviral conjunctivitis often occurs in epidemics in schools

■ Risk Factors

- Upper respiratory infection, community, or contact exposure

■ Etiology

- Usually bacterial, only 20% of cases are viral
- Common causes:
  - Bacterial: *H. influenzae, S. pneumoniae, N. gonorrhoeae, Moraxella catarrhalis, S. aureus, Haemophilus aegyptius*
  - Viral: Adenovirus, HSV, influenza, measles, varicella, Epstein-Barr virus

■ **Pathogenesis**
- Direct contact with infected secretions (hand-eye contact)
- Organisms infiltrate conjunctival epithelium

■ **History/Physical Examination**
- Red eye, tearing, discharge, foreign body sensation, itching, crusting of eyelids
- Conjunctival injection, discharge, papillae, edema (chemosis), or follicles (lymphoid hyperplasia)
- Subconjunctival hemorrhages

■ **Additional Studies**
- Mild conjunctivitis, diagnosis is made based on history and physical examination
- Acute severe, recurrent, or chronic conjunctivitis with poor response to therapy, perform cultures

■ **Differential Diagnosis**
- Blepharoconjunctivitis, allergic conjunctivitis, foreign body, trauma, chemical irritation, drug reaction, nasolacrimal duct obstruction, iritis, episcleritis, or scleritis

■ **Management**
- Bacterial conjunctivitis: Empiric ophthalmic antibiotics (trimethoprim/polymyxin B or quinolone)
- Viral conjunctivitis:
  - Herpes simplex conjunctivitis: Ophthalmic antiviral drops (vidarabine, trifluridine, idoxuridine). May require corneal debridement
  - Herpes zoster with conjunctivitis (rare): Systemic acyclovir; add steroids for iritis
  - Primary varicella infection with conjunctivitis: Ophthalmic trimethoprim/polymyxin B or fluoroquinolones to prevent superinfection
  - Other forms of viral conjunctivitis: Consider ophthalmic antibiotics to prevent bacterial superinfection

■ **Complications**
- Dry eyes, subconjunctival scarring, keratitis, and entropion

Endophthalmitis

- Infection of intraocular structures

■ Epidemiology

- In children, usually posttraumatic. In adults, 70% postoperative

■ Risk Factors

- Penetrating trauma, retained intraocular foreign body
- Intraocular surgery, especially if loss of vitreous, violation of posterior capsule, poor wound closure
- Infection of a filtering bleb after glaucoma surgery
- Systemic infection

■ Etiology

- Bacterial: Usually *S. epidermidis, S. pneumoniae, S. aureus, Propionibacterium acnes*
- Bacterial: Occasionally *P. aeruginosa, H. influenzae, Proteus* spp.
- In chronic postoperative endophthalmitis, *P. acnes* most common
- Fungal: *Candida albicans*
- Parasitic: *Toxocara canis, Toxoplasma gondii*

■ Pathogenesis

- Exogenous endophthalmitis: Direct inoculation through surgical or accidental trauma
- Endogenous endophthalmitis: Hematogenous spread from distant infection

■ History/Physical Examination

- Eye pain and redness, blurred vision, strabismus, recent trauma or surgery
- Reduced visual acuity, conjunctival injection, chemosis, vitritis, retinal periphlebitis, uveitis, hypopyon, leukocoria

■ Additional Studies

- Obtain aqueous and vitreous specimens by aspiration with an automated suction catheter
- Send for bacterial, fungal, and viral cultures and Gram and giemsa stains

■ Differential Diagnosis

- Severe uveitis, retinoblastoma, neuroblastoma, Langerhans cell histiocytosis, leukemia, lymphoma, metastatic tumor

■ Management

- Extrapolated from adult experience due to the paucity of published pediatric reports

- Bacterial endophthalmitis:
  - Intravitreal therapy with amikacin, ceftazidime plus vancomycin, or gentamicin (usually only one dose)
  - Systemic therapy with vancomycin plus gentamicin, amikacin, or ceftazidime
  - Topical cycloplegic agents (atropine)
  - Alter antibiotic therapy based on culture results. Consider systemic and topical steroids if no fungal infection
  - Vitrectomy may be considered in eyes with poor vision at presentation
- Fungal endophthalmitis
  - Aqueous and vitreous sampling as above, plus amphotericin B
- Parasitic endophthalmitis
  - Topical, periocular, or systemic steroids are used to manage inflammation in toxocariasis
  - For active toxoplasmosis: pyrimethamine, folinic acid, sulfadiazine with or without prednisone

▓ Complications
- Blindness and damage to all structures of the eye

Orbital and Periorbital Cellulitis

- Periorbital (preseptal) cellulitis: Infection of the skin and soft tissues anterior to the orbital septum
- Orbital cellulitis: Infection of the tissues posterior to the orbital septum

▓ Epidemiology/Risk Factors
- Periorbital cellulitis: Trauma, skin infection, chalazion, dacryocystitis, upper respiratory infection
- Orbital cellulitis: Chronic sinusitis, trauma, systemic infection

▓ Etiology
- Periorbital cellulitis: *S. aureus, S. pneumoniae, H. influenzae*
- Orbital cellulitis: *S. aureus, S. pneumoniae, Streptococcus pyogenes*, anaerobic cocci, *Prevotella* spp., *Fusobacterium* spp., *Veillonella* spp.
- Older children have an increased prevalence of anaerobes
- Few cases of *H. influenzae* since the introduction of the *H. influenzae* type B vaccine
- Fungal orbital cellulitis (mucormycosis) is uncommon; occurs in patients with ketoacidosis or immunosuppression

▓ Pathogenesis
- Periorbital cellulitis: Direct spread from nearby skin or lacrimal drainage system via the puncta

- 75% to 85% of cases of orbital cellulitis are related to sinusitis
- Factors predisposing to orbital extension of sinusitis
  - Natural bony dehiscences (lamina papyracea) exist in walls of ethmoid and sphenoid sinuses
  - Valveless orbital veins allow communication via blood flow of sinuses and orbits

■ **History**

- Red or swollen eyelids, headache, periorbital skin trauma, chronic sinus infection, upper respiratory infection

■ **Physical Examination**

- Periorbital cellulitis: Eyelid edema and erythema, mild conjunctival injection, normal extraocular movements, periorbital skin trauma
- Orbital cellulitis: Eyelid edema and erythema, proptosis, papillary disturbances, restricted extraocular movements, decreased visual acuity

■ **Additional Studies**

- Blood cultures
- Evaluation of cases presenting with orbital signs:
  - Orbital CT scan to evaluate for abscess or subperiosteal elevation
  - Cultures of blood and sinus aspirates (when possible)

■ **Differential Diagnosis**

- Periorbital cellulitis: Allergic reaction, trauma, angioneurotic edema, thyroid-related eye disease
- Orbital cellulitis: Orbital trauma, rhabdomyosarcoma, ruptured dermoid cyst, carotid cavernous fistula, thyroid eye disease

■ **Management**

- Periorbital cellulitis:
  - Hospitalize children under age 2 for IV antibiotics (ampicillin-sulbactam or cefotaxime IV)
  - Consider PO antibiotics in children younger than 2 years (amoxicillin-clavulanate, clindamycin)
  - If no improvement after 24 hours or if apparent worsening, obtain CT scan of the orbits
- Orbital cellulitis:
  - Hospitalize all children for IV antibiotics (ampicillin-sulbactam IV). Other options: Cefotaxime, cefuroxime, ceftriaxone, clindamycin, or ticarcillin-clavulanate

- CT scan of the orbits to detect abscess or foreign body
- Culture results should be used to tailor antibiotic therapy
- Gram stain and culture of surgical specimen (when available)
- Indications for surgery:
  - Ophthalmoplegia with visual loss
  - Subperiosteal abscess, globe displacement, or intraconal involvement with disease progression after 24 hours of antibiotic therapy

■ **Complications**

- Ocular sequelae: Compressive optic neuropathy, extraocular muscle scarring, neurotropic or ulcerative keratitis, secondary glaucoma, septic optic neuritis or uveitis, thromboembolic retinal disease
- Intracranial sequelae: Brain or epidural/subdural abscess, cavernous sinus thrombosis, meningitis

7

Central Nervous System Infections

Jeffrey M. Bergelson, MD

Meningitis

• Inflammation of the meninges surrounding the brain

■ Epidemiology

• Bacterial meningitis is most common in infants and young children
• Dramatic decrease in incidence after immunization with *Haemophilus influenzae* type B (Hib) and 7-valent pneumococcal vaccines
• *Neisseria meningitidis* meningitis occurs shortly after exposure to the organism
• Enteroviral meningitis is seen in summer and fall

■ Risk Factors

• Immune deficiency (hypogammaglobulinemia, splenic dysfunction, complement deficiency); anatomic abnormality (CSF fistula)

■ Etiology (Table 7-1)

• Viral: Enteroviruses most common (ECHO, coxsackie); also insect-borne viruses (e.g., equine encephalitis, West Nile); mumps; herpes simplex; others
• In immunocompromised patients: *Listeria, Cryptococcus neoformans*
• Other infectious causes include syphilis, endemic fungi (e.g., histoplasma), amebae
• Parameningeal: Infections contiguous to the meninges (brain abscess, sinusitis, epidural abscess) can cause meningeal inflammation with negative cultures
• Noninfectious: Vasculitis (e.g., lupus), tumors, intrathecal injections, drugs [e.g., trimethoprim-sulfamethoxazole (Bactrim), nonsteroidal anti-inflammatory drugs, intravenous immunoglobulin]

▉ TABLE 7-1 Common Causes of Meningitis by Age

Neonates	6 weeks–Adulthood
Group B *Streptococcus*	*Streptococcus pneumoniae*
E. coli (and other gram-negative bacilli)	*Neisseria meningitidis*
Listeria monocytogenes	*Haemophilus influenzae*[a]
Enterovirus	Enterovirus
Herpes simplex[b]	*Borrelia burgdorferi*
	Mycobacterium tuberculosis

[a] *Haemophilus influenzae* type b meningitis is unusual in the neonate.
[b] Herpes simplex encephalitis should be considered in newborns with aseptic meningitis.

▉ Pathogenesis

- Major bacterial pathogens colonize the throat, then spread through the bloodstream to the meninges
- Contiguous infection or trauma can also deliver bacteria to the CSF space

▉ History

- Fever, headache, vomiting, convulsions, altered mental status, photophobia
- Young babies may show nonspecific signs of sepsis (e.g., poor feeding, somnolence)
- Tuberculous meningitis develops subacutely (usually over a week or more)
- Ask about exposures, travel, pretreatment with antibiotics, immunologic problems

▉ Physical Examination

- Stiff neck (not seen in infants): Kernig sign (resistance to extension of the knee); Brudzinski sign (involuntary flexion of the hip/leg when the neck is flexed)
- Bulging fontanelle in infants; irritability
- Focal neurologic signs suggest intracranial complication [perform CT/MRI before lumbar puncture (LP)]
- Petechial or purpuric rash in meningococcal or rickettsial infection

▉ Additional Studies

- LP and spinal fluid examination (Table 7-2)
- CSF culture, blood culture
- Complete blood count, electrolytes, glucose

■ TABLE 7-2 Cerebrospinal Fluid Evaluation

	WBC	Glucose	Protein	Gram Stain
Bacterial	Neutrophils: 100s–1000s	Low [a]	High	Positive
Viral	Mononuclear: hundreds	Normal	Slightly increased	Negative
TB	Mononuclear; hundreds	Low	High	Negative
Cryptococcal	Mononuclear: few–100s	Low	Normal or high	Negative
Parameningeal	Mononuclear: few	Normal	High	Negative

[a] Less than 50% serum glucose.

- CT or MRI if focal findings, seizures, or suspected intracranial complication
- In special circumstances: Purified protein derivative (PPD), acid-fast bacillus (AFB) culture, fungal culture, cryptococcal antigen, enteroviral or herpes simplex (HSV) polymerase chain reaction (PCR), viral cultures

■ **Differential Diagnosis**

- Fever and neurologic findings: Meningitis, encephalitis, intracranial abscess
- Although "aseptic meningitis" (lymphocytic pleocytosis and negative bacterial cultures) is often caused by enteroviruses, the findings are not specific
  - In newborns, always exclude herpes encephalitis
  - If symptoms worsen or persist, consider parameningeal or tuberculous infection

■ **Management**

- Maintain oxygenation and circulation; control intracranial pressure
- Direct initial antibiotic therapy at most common organisms (Table 7-1)
  - Empiric: In neonates, ampicillin plus cefotaxime (if gram-negative rods on Gram stain, use carbapenem plus aminoglycoside). In older children, use vancomycin plus cefotaxime (or ceftriaxone). For cephalosporin-allergic patients, consider ciprofloxacin, meropenem, or rifampin.
  - Definitive (Table 7-3)
  - Add coverage–but don't reduce it–based on Gram stain results

▓ TABLE 7-3 Definitive Therapy for Meningitis[a]		
Organism	**Antibiotic**	**Duration**
Group B *Streptococcus*	Penicillin ± gentamicin	2–3 wk
E. coli	Cefotaxime or imipenem/meropenem	3–6 wk
Streptococcus pneumoniae	If sensitive to penicillin: penicillin	10–14 d
	If sensitive to cefotaxime, resistant to penicillin: cefotaxime	
	If resistant to cefotaxime and penicillin, but sensitive to vancomycin: cefotaxime + vancomycin ± rifampin	
Neisseria meningitidis	Penicillin (or cefotaxime)[b]	7 d
Haemophilus influenzae	Ampicillin (if sensitive) or cefotaxime	7 d
Listeria monocytogenes	Ampicillin ± gentamicin	2–3 wk
	Alternative: TMP-SMX	

[a] Should be adjusted according to sensitivity testing.
[b] In the United States, meningococci are routinely sensitive to penicillin; in Africa and Europe, penicillin-resistant isolates are encountered.

- Length of therapy: *S. pneumoniae*, 10 to 14 days; *N. meningitidis*, 5 to 7 days; Hib, 7 days
- Antibiotic prophylaxis for close contacts of patients with meningococcal meningitis

▓ Complications

- Complications of bacterial meningitis include intracranial infection (subdural empyema, brain abscess), cerebral infarction, hyponatremia, and disseminated infection (arthritis, pneumonia)
- Outcomes of pneumococcal meningitis: mortality 8%; motor deficit 25%; hearing loss 32%
- No expected long-term sequelae after enteroviral meningitis

Encephalitis

- Inflammation of the brain parenchyma; often accompanied by meningeal involvement

▓ Epidemiology

- Herpes simplex virus (HSV) encephalitis: In neonates, perinatal acquisition usually after primary maternal genital infection (see Chapter 17). In older children, HSV encephalitis is most commonly associated with reactivation

- Viral encephalitis often transmitted by mosquitoes (may be associated with outbreaks of illness in animal populations)
- Postinfectious encephalitis often occurs after relatively minor respiratory infections (including mycoplasma) and sometimes after vaccinations
- Cat scratch encephalitis after contact with kittens
- Cysticercosis, caused by the pork tapeworm, is common outside the United States; patients present with seizures

■ Risk Factors

- Most patients have no predisposing illness

■ Etiology

- Viruses: Herpes simplex, insect-borne (Eastern and Western equine, California, La Crosse, West Nile, Japanese), rabies, enteroviruses, varicella, Epstein-Barr virus, others
- Bacteria: *Mycobacterium tuberculosis*, *Bartonella henselae* (cat scratch), *Listeria monocytogenes* (in immunocompromised patients)
- Parasites: *Toxoplasma gondii* (in immunocompromised), *Cysticercus*

■ Pathogenesis

- Viral infection of the brain parenchyma causes cellular damage and provokes inflammatory response
- Postinfectious encephalitis is believed to be immune mediated

■ History

- Fever, headache, altered mental status, convulsions
- Ask about mosquito and animal bites, bat exposure, travel, exposure to tuberculosis, recent vaccinations

■ Physical Examination

- Neurologic exam: Focality makes HSV more likely. Extremity weakness suggests West Nile virus
- General exam: Evidence of systemic illness. Local adenopathy may suggest cat-scratch disease

■ Additional Studies

- CSF evaluation
  - Viral encephalitis most often causes mononuclear cell pleocytosis; Eastern equine encephalitis causes neutrophilic pleocytosis
  - PCR for enteroviruses, HSV, and some arboviruses

- Magnetic resonance image may show focal involvement or evidence of demyelination
  - HSV in adult typically affects temporal lobe
- Electroencephalogram may show evidence of focality
- Arbovirus serology, including West Nile virus
- Tuberculin skin testing (PPD)
- Cat scratch serology and PCR if suspected

■ Differential Diagnosis

- Bacterial meningitis typically causes neutrophilic pleocytosis; viral meningitis usually does not cause marked CNS dysfunction
- Vasculitis; tumor; genetic and metabolic causes of cerebral dysfunction

■ Management

- Acyclovir for possible HSV encephalitis
  - In neonates: 60 mg/kg/d, divided into three doses, for 21 days
  - In children and adults: 1500 mg/m^2, divided into three doses, for 14 to 21 days
- Specific therapies for most other viruses are not available
- Steroids for documented demyelinating illness
- Control of seizures

■ Complications

- Patients with viral encephalitis may have good recovery or may have persistent cognitive and motor defects
  - HSV, Eastern equine encephalitis often have poor prognosis
  - Cat-scratch encephalitis has good prognosis

Subdural Empyema and Epidural Abscess

- Intracranial infection may be confined to the spaces between the dura and the inner table of the skull or spinal column (epidural abscess), or between the meninges and dura (subdural empyema)

■ Risk Factors

- Intracranial empyema: Bacterial meningitis (subdural), otitis or sinusitis (subdural or epidural)
- Spinal epidural abscess may occur as a complication of vertebral osteomyelitis or as a consequence of bacteremia

■ Etiology

- When it occurs as a complication of bacterial meningitis, subdural empyema is often caused by *Streptococcus pneumoniae* or *H. influenzae*; when sinusitis or otitis spread to the subdural or epidural space, consider anaerobes, gram-negative aerobes, *Streptococcus milleri*, and *Staphylococcus aureus*
- Spinal epidural abscess is commonly caused by *S. aureus*, but gram-negative organisms may also be involved; tuberculous osteomyelitis should be considered

■ History

- Intracranial: Fever, headache
- Spinal: Back pain

■ Physical Examination

- Intracranial infection: Fever, meningeal signs, papilledema, focal neurologic signs; epidural abscess rarely causes increased intracranial pressure
- Spinal epidural abscess: Fever, local tenderness, motor and sensory loss

■ Additional Studies

- CT or MRI is essential
- Gram stain and culture of abscess fluid
- Blood culture
- LP often shows pleocytosis with negative cultures
- Place PPD and stain CSF for AFB if subacute or chronic infection

■ Differential Diagnosis

- Fever/headache: Meningitis, brain abscess, encephalitis, sinusitis
- Spinal epidural abscess: Tumors, transverse myelitis, vertebral osteomyelitis
- Aseptic meningitis associated with bacteremia: Search for parameningeal abscess

■ Management

- Surgical drainage
- Antibiotics:
  - Intracranial: Vancomycin plus cefotaxime/ceftriaxone plus metronidazole
  - Spinal: Vancomycin plus cefotaxime/ceftriaxone/ceftazidime

■ Complications

- Intracranial: Subdural empyema may cause herniation. Both subdural and epidural empyema may cause thrombosis of cerebral veins and venous sinuses
- Spinal: Spinal cord compression and paralysis

Brain Abscess

■ Risk Factors
- Right-to-left vascular shunts: Cyanotic congenital heart disease
- Neonatal meningitis, especially *Citrobacter koseri*
- Chronic sinusitis, otitis, dental abscess, lung abscess
- Penetrating trauma or craniotomy

■ Etiology
- Bacteria: Viridans streptococci (especially *S. milleri*), anaerobes, *S. aureus*, occasionally gram-negative aerobic bacilli (especially after trauma, craniotomy, or with chronic otitis/mastoiditis)
- In immunocompromised patients: Fungi (especially aspergillus), *T. gondii*, *L. monocytogenes*, *Nocardia species*

■ Pathogenesis
- May occur as a result of bacteremia, or as an extension of sinusitis or otitis

■ History/Physical Examination
- Headache, fever, altered mental status
- Altered mental status, papilledema, focal neurologic signs

■ Additional Studies
- Head CT or MRI
- Blood culture
- Chest X-ray
- Culture of abscess fluid (lumbar puncture is contraindicated; risk of herniation)

■ Differential Diagnosis
- Brain abscess must be differentiated from other CNS infections (meningitis, encephalitis) and from other intracranial mass lesions

■ Management
- Control of intracranial pressure
- Aspiration or surgical drainage, especially for large lesions with mass effect
  - Early cerebritis or small inaccessible lesions may resolve with medical therapy
- Antibiotic therapy
  - Empiric regimen: Cefotaxime/ceftriaxone plus metronidazole (± vancomycin)
  - If associated with otitis or mastoiditis: Replace cefotaxime with ceftazidime

- After trauma or neurosurgery: vancomycin plus ceftazidime
- Adjust once culture results are known
- Prolonged treatment (more than 6 weeks) often necessary

■ Complications
- Seizures; cerebral herniation; rupture into ventricles may cause acute decompensation

Ventricular Shunt Infections

■ Etiology
- Common: *S. epidermidis*
- Less common: *Propionibacterium acnes*, *S. aureus*, enteric gram-negative bacilli
- Rare: *Candida* species

■ Pathogenesis
- Bacteria of low virulence colonize the skin. Shunts may become contaminated at the time of placement
- Erosion of skin over shunt or perforation of abdominal viscus causes late infection

■ History
- Fever, shunt dysfunction, redness of skin overlying shunt, abdominal symptoms

■ Physical Examination
- Look for signs of increased intracranial pressure, meningeal inflammation, inflammation along the path of shunt, peritoneal signs

■ Additional Studies
- Aspirate shunt fluid: Culture and Gram stain; mild pleocytosis may occur without infection
- MRI or CT to rule out abscess if response to therapy is delayed

■ Differential Diagnosis
- Shunt infection may mimic shunt dysfunction without infection

■ Management
- Combined medical and surgical treatment:
  1) Remove shunt, insert intraventricular drain
  2) Treat with antibiotics until cultures are negative
  3) Replace shunt and treat several days more

- Empiric antibiotics: Intravenous vancomycin (± intrathecal gentamicin); if severely ill, add intravenous broad gram-negative coverage as well
  - CSF penetration poor in the absence of inflammation
  - Intrathecal vancomycin administration may be necessary if response is poor
  - Some centers use oral trimethoprim-sulfamethoxazole (TMP-SMX) plus rifampin
- Longer treatment may be necessary for frank meningitis, abscess, or cellulitis

■ Complications

- Shunt infections generally resolve with appropriate therapy
- Some patients suffer repeated infections
- Distal infection (e.g., peritonitis) may occur

8 Upper Respiratory Tract Infections

Susmita Pati, MD, MPH, Nicholas Tsarouhas, MD,
and Samir S. Shah, MD

Pharyngitis

■ Epidemiology
- Generally in children older than 3 years. Peaks in late winter/ early spring

■ Risk Factors
- Day care attendance; crowded living conditions

■ Etiology
- Bacterial: Group A *Streptococcus* (GAS), Group C and G streptococci, *Arcanobacterium haemolyticum*, *Neisseria gonorrhoeae*, *Corynebacterium diphtheriae*, *Mycoplasma pneumoniae*
- Viral: Adenovirus, Epstein-Barr virus (EBV), influenza, parainfluenza, enteroviruses
- Most cases viral but 15–20% due to GAS

■ Pathogenesis
- Inhalation of organisms in large droplets or by direct contact with respiratory secretions
- Incubation period is 2 to 5 days for GAS pharyngitis and 28 to 42 days for EBV

■ History
- Fever, throat pain, trouble swallowing, hoarseness, refusal to eat
- GAS: Headache, abdominal pain

■ Physical Examination
- Erythema of pharynx with or without exudates
- GAS: Tender anterior cervical adenopathy, palatal petechiae, or "strawberry tongue"
- EBV: Exudative pharyngitis, generalized adenopathy, hepatosplenomegaly, amoxicillin rash

- *A. haemolyticum*: Scarlatiniform rash (prominent on extensor surfaces) usually in teenagers

■ **Additional Studies**

- GAS rapid antigen detection studies: Sensitivity greater than 80%; specificity greater than 95%
- GAS culture: "Gold standard"; recommended when rapid studies are negative
- "Monospot" (heterophile antibody) test: EBV diagnosis, but not reliable if patient is younger than 5 years
- EBV titers: "Gold standard"; necessary to diagnose EBV in children younger than 5 years
- Atypical lymphocytosis and mild thrombocytopenia: Classic CBC findings with EBV

■ **Differential Diagnosis**

- Stomatitis, peritonsillar or retropharyngeal abscess, dental abscess

■ **Management**

- GAS: 1) Penicillin V (first-line oral agent); 2) benzathine penicillin (single IM injection obviates compliance issues); 3) amoxicillin (common, practical alternative to oral penicillin); 4) other options include clindamycin, cephalosporins, and macrolides
- *N. gonorrhoeae*: IM ceftriaxone (one dose)
- EBV: 1) supportive care; 2) avoid contact sports until splenomegaly resolves; and 3) steroids if impending airway obstruction from tonsillar enlargement

■ **Complications**

- GAS infections: 1) Suppurative (peritonsillar or retropharyngeal abscess, cervical lymphadenitis); 2) nonsuppurative including rheumatic fever (prevented if therapy started within 9 days of symptom onset) and glomerulonephritis (therapy does not alter risk)

Peritonsillar and Retropharyngeal Abscess

- Peritonsillar abscess ("quinsy"): Purulent collection in the tonsillar fossa
- Retropharyngeal abscess: Infection of the lymph nodes found in the potential space between the posterior pharyngeal wall and the prevertebral fascia

■ Epidemiology/Risk Factors

- Peritonsillar abscess: Usually occurs in adolescents but occasionally in younger children.
- Retropharyngeal abscess: Usually in children younger than 5 years, as these nodes atrophy and disappear later in childhood

■ Etiology

- Most common: GAS; α-hemolytic streptococci; oral anaerobes; *Staphylococcus aureus*

■ Pathogenesis

- Peritonsillar abscess: Infectious tonsillopharyngitis progresses from cellulitis to abscess
- Retropharyngeal abscess: Lymphatics drain nasopharynx/posterior sinuses/adenoids
  - Purulent infections in these regions spread to retropharynx by lymphatic drainage.
  - Retropharyngeal lymph node inflammation followed by necrosis leads to abscess
  - Rarely, infection caused by penetrating neck injury or extension of cervical osteomyelitis

■ History

- Fever, sore throat, dysphagia, drooling, refusal to eat
- Peritonsillar abscess: Also trismus, muffled ("hot-potato") voice, unilateral neck or ear pain
- Retropharyngeal abscess: Also neck pain or stiffness

■ Physical Examination

Peritonsillar Abscess
- Unilateral peritonsillar fullness; uvular deviation; bulging of posterior superior soft palate; palpable fluctuance of palatal swelling
- Erythematous and edematous pharynx, enlarged and exudative tonsils, cervical adenopathy
- Occasionally torticollis

Retropharyngeal Abscess
- Neck pain especially with extension; head maintained in neutral position; torticollis
- Occasionally meningismus or stridor (less than 5%)

■ Additional Studies

- GAS throat studies: Often positive (see "Pharyngitis")
- Gram stain and culture of aspirate specimen from abscess

Peritonsillar Abscess
- CT scan or ultrasound: Differentiate peritonsillar cellulitis from peritonsillar abscess

Retropharyngeal Abscess
- Lateral neck X-ray: Initial diagnostic study of choice; suspect abscess if, at level of C2/C3, the prevertebral soft-tissue space is more than half the adjacent vertebral body diameter
- CT scan: Confirms diagnosis, delineates extent, and distinguishes abscess from cellulitis

■ **Differential Diagnosis**
- Stridor: Croup, tracheitis, epiglottitis, foreign body, angioedema, cystic hygroma (infected)
- Torticollis: Pharyngitis, cervical adenitis, vertebral osteomyelitis, Lemierre syndrome
- Retropharyngeal mass: Neoplasm, hemangioma, ectopic thyroid, congenital myxedema, lymphadenopathy (e.g., Kawasaki disease, histiocytosis)

■ **Management**

Peritonsillar Abscess
- Otorhinolaryngology consultation
- Drain true abscesses via either needle aspiration or surgical incision
- First-line antibiotic therapy: Intravenous penicillin
- Alternative antibiotic therapy: Clindamycin, oxacillin, cefazolin, or ampicillin-sulbactam
- Antibiotic course: 10–14 days. Oral antibiotics when fever/peritonsillar swelling subside

Retropharyngeal Abscess
- Antibiotics, otorhinolaryngology consultation, and, in most cases, operative drainage
- If CT reveals inflammatory changes (phlegmon) but no clear abscess, treat with antibiotics and consider repeat imaging in 24 to 72 hours if insufficient clinical improvement
- First-line antibiotics: Ampicillin-sulbactam
- Alternative: Cefotaxime plus metronidazole or monotherapy with clindamycin (especially if high MRSA prevalence)

■ **Complications**

Peritonsillar or Retropharyngeal Abscess
- Upper airway obstruction, dehydration

Retropharyngeal Abscess
- Extension to carotid sheath (carotid artery, internal jugular vein, vagus nerve)
- Extension posteriorly causing atlantoaxial dislocation
- Spontaneous rupture causing aspiration, asphyxiation, or mediastinitis

Croup

- Croup syndrome (laryngotracheitis or laryngotracheobronchitis): Spectrum of diseases causing upper airway obstruction

■ Epidemiology
- Usually occurs in late fall and winter, but sporadic cases throughout the year
- Peak incidence at 18 months (typical range, 1 to 6 years)

■ Risk Factors/Etiology
- Common: Parainfluenza types 1, 2, and 3
- Less common: Influenza viruses A, B
- Rare: Respiratory syncytial virus (RSV), adenovirus, measles

■ Pathogenesis
- Virus-induced inflammation of trachea and vocal cords
- Subglottic (narrowest part of a child's upper airway) tracheal edema restricts airflow

■ History/Physical Examination
- Dry, barking cough that worsens at night; hoarse voice; inspiratory stridor
- Antecedent upper respiratory infection (URI)
- Hypoxia only with severe croup
- Inspiratory stridor (from turbulent airflow); hoarse voice (from vocal cord edema); coryza, mildly inflamed pharynx

■ Additional Studies
- 50% of cases reveal abnormal neck radiographs
  - Posteroanterior view: Tapered subglottic narrowing ("steeple sign")
  - Lateral view: Overdistention of hypopharynx

■ Differential Diagnosis
- Infectious: Acute epiglottitis; retropharyngeal/peritonsillar abscess; bacterial tracheitis; infectious mononucleosis; laryngeal diphtheria

- Other: Angioneurotic edema; subglottic stenosis; tracheomalacia; foreign body aspiration

■ Management

- **Cool mist treatment** (Caution: May intensify bronchospasm)
  - Mechanism of action: soothes inflamed mucosa, decreases viscosity of tracheal secretions; may activate larynx mechanoreceptors to produce reflex slowing of respiratory flow rate
  - No clinical trials have demonstrated efficacy
- **Corticosteroids**: For any patient with increased work of breathing
  - Mechanism of action: Decreases laryngeal mucosal edema via anti-inflammatory action
  - Dexamethasone 0.6 mg/kg PO or IM (max 10 mg), clinical improvement in 4 to 6 hours
  - For mild-moderate croup, dexamethasone 0.15–0.30 mg/kg is effective
  - Nebulized budesonide (2 mg): Unclear role since dexamethasone easier to administer
- **Nebulized epinephrine**: For severe or worsening respiratory distress
  - Mechanism of action: α-agonist capillary arteriole constriction decreases mucosal edema
  - Dose: 0.25–0.75 mL of 2.25% racemic epinephrine solution in 2.5 mL of normal saline
  - "Rebound" phenomenon (2 to 4 hours after treatment) rare if dexamethasone also given
  - Hospitalization unnecessary if after 3 to 4 hours: 1) no stridor at rest, 2) normal air entry, 3) normal color, 4) normal level of consciousness, and 5) received dexamethasone
- **Helium-oxygen therapy** (usually 70% He:30% O_2): Helium (low-density and low-viscosity gas) improves laminar gas flow and decreases mechanical work of breathing
  - Endotracheal intubation may be required for severe croup

■ Complications

- Bacterial superinfection (*S. aureus*, *S. pyogenes*, *S. pneumoniae*, and *H. influenzae*)

Otitis Media

- Otitis media (OM): Inflammation of mucosa lining the middle ear
  - Acute otitis media (AOM): Acute middle ear inflammation with local or systemic illness

- Recurrent AOM: Less than three episodes in 6 months, or four or more episodes in 1 year
- Chronic suppurative OM: Purulent drainage from perforated tympanic membrane more than 6 weeks

■ Epidemiology

- 90% of children have at least one episode of AOM by 2 years of age; 50% have three or more episodes by age 3. Incidence greatest between 6 and 18 months of age.

■ Risk Factors

- Congenital: Craniofacial anomaly; immunodeficiency; dysfunctional cilia; male sex
- Acquired: Allergy; bottle-feeding; day care attendance; siblings; tobacco smoke exposure
- Risk of **recurrent** AOM is higher if the first episode occurs at age 6 months or younger

■ Etiology

- *S. pneumoniae* (35% to 48%); Nontypeable *H. influenzae* (20% to 29%); *Moraxella catarrhalis* (12% to 23%); GAS (less than 5%); *S. aureus* (less than 5%)
- Viruses cause 10% to 40% of middle ear effusions in AOM
- Chronic suppurative OM: Mixed flora including *Pseudomonas aeruginosa* and *S. aureus*

■ Pathogenesis

- Eustachian tube dysfunction caused by viral URI or other factors (see "Risk Factors")
- Tube dysfunction leads to negative middle ear pressure; middle ear fluid accumulates; bacterial infection follows

■ History/Physical Examination

- Ear pain, pulling at ear, otorrhea, fever, crying, sleep disturbance
- Examination of tympanic membrane: 1) Decreased mobility by pneumatic otoscopy; 2) red or yellow color; 3) bulging or thickened ; 4) poorly visualized landmarks; 5) dull light reflex; 6) perforation with drainage

■ Additional Studies

- Tympanometry confirms middle ear effusion when pneumatic otoscopy is impossible
- Indications for tympanocentesis: 1) Relieve severe pain; 2) confirm pathogens in neonates or immunocompromised children; 3) failed antibiotic therapy; 4) treatment for mastoiditis

■ **Differential Diagnosis**
- Retained foreign body, otitis externa, traumatic tympanic membrane perforation, pharyngitis with referred pain, basilar skull fracture, tumors

■ **Management**
- AOM (Based on AAP recommendations. Pediatrics 2004; 113:1451–1465)
  - Pain control with acetaminophen or ibuprofen. In children older than 5 years consider topical benzocaine
  - For age less than 2 years and for those with severe otalgia or fever ≥39°C, treat with antibiotics (see below)
  - For age older than or equal to 2 years, consider initial observation without antibiotics if illness is not severe or diagnosis is uncertain. Then treat if no improvement within 48–72 hours. (If observation option exercised, ensure follow-up and availability of antibiotics if necessary.)
  - First-line therapy: High-dose amoxicillin (90 mg/kg/d)
  - Duration of therapy: 5 days but treat 10 days if child younger than 2 years or with underlying medical conditions, recurrent AOM, or chronic suppurative OM
  - Alternative for treatment failure, amoxicillin allergy, and recurrent AOM: Amoxicillin-clavulanate (high dose) or cefuroxime, cefdinir, clindamycin, ceftriaxone, or azithromycin
- Recurrent AOM
  - Treat as above followed by prophylaxis with sulfisoxazole or amoxicillin for 3 to 6 months
- Asymptomatic middle ear effusions routinely follow AOM (not considered treatment failure)
  - 40% at 1 month after AOM; 20% at 2 months; and 10% at 3 months
  - Effusions usually sterile so antibiotic management of OME not recommended
- Chronic suppurative OM
  - 7 to 14 days of ototopical antibiotics; consider oral antibiotics as for AOM
- Indications for tympanostomy tubes: 1) Chronic OME (more than 3 months) and associated conductive hearing loss greater than 15 dB; 2) failed chemoprophylaxis for recurrent AOM; 3) tympanic membrane retraction with ossicular erosion or cholesteatoma formation.

■ **Complications**
- Middle ear: Cholesteatoma, conductive hearing loss, facial nerve paralysis, ossicular damage, tympanic membrane perforation

- Temporal bone: Mastoiditis, petrositis
- Inner ear: Labyrinthitis, neurosensory hearing loss
- Intracranium: Intracranial abscess, lateral sinus thrombosis, meningitis, otitic hydrocephalus

Mastoiditis

- Infection of mastoid air cell system (with or without bone destruction) caused by middle ear suppuration. May be acute or chronic (symptoms more than 6 weeks)

■ Epidemiology/Risk Factors

- Usually age less than 5 years
- Risk factors: Viral infections, ciliary dysfunction, and immunodeficiency

■ Etiology

- Acute mastoiditis
  - Common: *S. pneumoniae, S. aureus, S. pyogenes, H. influenzae*
  - Less common: *P. aeruginosa, Proteus* species
- Chronic mastoiditis
  - *S. aureus, P. aeruginosa*, other gram-negative bacilli, and anaerobes

■ Pathogenesis

- Middle ear infection spreads to mastoid
- Serous then purulent material accumulates within mastoid cavities
- Thin bony septa between mastoid air cells may be destroyed
- Potential dissection of pus into adjacent areas (see "Complications")

■ History/Physical Examination

- Recent OM, ear discharge, ear pain, hearing loss, or fever
- Auricle displaced: *Downward* and outward in infants *but upward* and outward in older child
- Mastoid swelling, tenderness, and erythema; blunted postauricular sulcus
- Drainage fistula may be present
- Tympanic membrane inflamed or perforated
- Chronic mastoiditis: Middle ear granulation tissue or polypoid formations

■ Additional Studies

- Contrast-enhanced head CT to define extent of disease

■ **Differential Diagnosis**

• Cellulitis, posterior auricular lymphadenitis

■ **Management**

• Acute mastoiditis
  - Myringotomy to drain middle ear and mastoid and to obtain culture data
  - Parenteral antibiotic treatment (cefotaxime, ceftriaxone, or ampicillin-sulbactam)
  - Mastoidectomy if fever and otalgia persist for more than 48 hours or if infection progresses
• Chronic mastoiditis
  - Antibiotic therapy as above plus myringotomy and mastoidectomy

■ **Complications**

• Meningitis, epidural or subdural abscess, otogenic extradural brain abscess, lateral sinus thrombosis, or facial nerve palsy
• Extension medially to petrous air cells (petrositis)
• Extension through mastoid tip (sternocleidomastoid abscess, a.k.a., Bezold abscess)
• Extension through digastric groove (digastric triangle abscess, a.k.a., Citelli abscess)
• Retropharyngeal or parapharyngeal abscess

Sinusitis

• Defined as paranasal sinus inflammation
• Classification depends on duration of symptoms: Acute (less than 30 days); subacute (4 to 12 weeks); and chronic (more than 12 weeks)

■ **Epidemiology**

• Complicates 5% to 10% of URIs

■ **Risk Factors**

• Mucosal swelling: Viral URI, allergic inflammation, cystic fibrosis, immune disorders, immotile cilia, facial trauma, swimming, diving, rhinitis medicamentosa
• Mechanical obstruction: Choanal atresia, deviated septum, nasal polyps, foreign body, tumor, ethmoid bullae, encephalocele

■ **Etiology**

• Acute and subacute sinusitis
  - Bacterial: 30% to 40% *S. pneumoniae*; 20% *H. influenzae* (nontypeable); 20% *M. catarrhalis*
  - Viral: Adenovirus, parainfluenza, influenza, and rhinovirus

- Chronic sinusitis
  - Similar to acute sinusitis except more likely to have anaerobes, *S. aureus* (3%), enteric gram-negative rods (2%), and penicillin-resistant *S. pneumoniae*

■ Pathogenesis

- Sinus development
  - Maxillary and ethmoid sinuses form during third to fourth gestational month
  - Sphenoid sinuses pneumatize by age 5
  - Frontal sinuses start to develop at age 5 to 6 years but fully pneumatize during late adolescence
- Retention of paranasal sinus secretions due to obstructed ostia, impaired ciliary number/function, and altered viscosity of the secretions

■ History

Acute Sinusitis

- Persistent *and* nonimproving respiratory symptoms (10 days or more)
- Nasal discharge of *any* quality
- Daytime cough, halitosis, facial pain, headache, painless morning periorbital edema
- Fever, if present, is usually low grade
- Less common presentation: High fever (39.0°C), purulent nasal discharge

Chronic Sinusitis

- Nasal obstruction, cough, sore throat, postnasal drip
- Nasal discharge and headache are less common and fever is rare

■ Physical Examination

- Reproducible unilateral sinus pain on palpation
- Pressure over the body of maxillary and frontal sinuses
- Mild erythema and swelling of the nasal turbinates; "cobble-stoning" of posterior pharynx
- Sinus transillumination: Most useful if completely opaque or normal (sensitivity 50% to 75% in older children)

■ Additional Studies

- Diagnosis based on history and examination; radiologic imaging not routinely required
- Plain films: Diffuse opacification, mucosal thickening of at least 4 mm, or air-fluid levels

- Sinus/head CT useful in some situations: 1) Suspected complication of sinusitis, 2) persistent or recurrent symptoms, and 3) anticipated surgical intervention
- Indications for sinus aspiration: 1) Failure to respond to multiple antibiotic courses, 2) severe facial pain, 3) orbital or intracranial complications, and 4) immunocompromised host
  - Send for quantitative aerobic and anaerobic cultures, fungal cultures, and Gram stain

■ Differential Diagnosis

- Viral URI, adenoiditis, allergic rhinosinusitis

■ Management

- Acute or subacute bacterial sinusitis
  - Amoxicillin (45 mg/kg/d) for 10 to 14 days (maximum dose, 3 g/d)
  - Clinical improvement usually occurs within 48 to 72 hours
  - Alternative regimens: High-dose amoxicillin (80–90 mg/kg/d) or amoxicillin-clavulanate, cefuroxime axetil, cefpodoxime, azithromycin, clarithromycin, or levofloxacin
- Hospitalization for orbital or central nervous system complications
  - Empiric therapy: Cefotaxime, ceftriaxone, or ampicillin-sulbactam. Consider adding vancomycin (for methicillin-resistant *S. aureus*) or metronidazole (for anaerobes)
  - Ear-nose-throat and infectious diseases consultation and perhaps surgical drainage
- Adjuvant therapies: None routinely recommended
  - Hypertonic or isotonic saline nasal spray (inexpensive, occasionally beneficial)
  - Intranasal steroids beneficial to those with allergic precipitants
- Surgery for patients with chronic sinusitis not responding to maximal medical therapy

■ Complications

- Periorbital cellulitis, orbital cellulitis or abscess, optic neuritis
- Epidural/subdural empyema, meningitis, brain abscess
- Cavernous or sagittal sinus thrombosis
- Frontal (Pott puffy tumor) or maxillary osteomyelitis

Cervical Lymphadenitis

- Submental, submandibular, or superior cervical lymph node infection

■ Epidemiology

- Typically between ages 1 and 4 years

■ Risk Factors

- Contact with cats (*Bartonella henselae, Toxoplasma gondii, Pasteurella multocida, Yersinia pestis*) or rabbits (*Francisella tularensis*)
- Phagocyte defect (e.g., hyper-IgE)
- Dental caries predispose to anaerobic infection

■ Etiology

- Common: *S. aureus*, GAS, GBS (neonates)
- Less common: *B. henselae* (cat-scratch), nontuberculous mycobacteria (NTM), anaerobes
- Rare: *Mycobacterium tuberculosis, T. gondii, F. tularensis, P. multocida, Y. pestis*, gram-negative bacilli, *Nocardia* species

■ Pathogenesis

- Local infection in lymph node may follow hematogenous spread of systemic infection or lymphatic drainage of infected area

■ History

- Inquire about specific exposures, recent travel, dental problems, and systemic symptoms
- Inquire about symptoms associated with compression of adjacent neck structures

■ Physical Examination

- Bacterial: Unilateral, firm, tender, warm, overlying cellulitis, occasionally fluctuant
- *B. henselae*: Follows scratch/bite by 1 to 8 weeks, nontender, solitary large (more than 4 cm) node, no overlying discoloration or cellulitis, 25% with associated fever
- NTM: Gradual enlargement (weeks to months), minimal tenderness, overlying skin becomes violaceous as nodes soften and 10% drain spontaneously through sinus tract to skin
- *M. tuberculosis*: Gradual enlargement, nontender, firm, primary pulmonary focus in 30% to 70%

■ Additional Studies

- Consider CT or ultrasound of neck to detect suppurative nodes and extent of infection
- *B. henselae:* Serology (indirect fluorescent antibody) or polymerase chain reaction of serum or lymph node
- NTM: Tuberculin skin test usually 5 to 9 mm
- *M. tuberculosis*: Tuberculin skin test usually more than 15 mm; chest radiographic findings may include hilar adenopathy, cavitary lesion, or pleural effusion

■ **Differential Diagnosis**

- Miscellaneous lymphadenopathy: Kawasaki syndrome, PFAPA, sarcoid, Rosai-Dorfman (sinus histiocytosis with lymphadenopathy), Kikuchi-Fujimoto (histiocytic necrotizing lymphadenitis), Kimura disease, Castleman disease (giant lymph node hyperplasia)
- Congential: Thyroglossal duct cyst, branchial cleft cyst, dermoid cyst, goiter, lymphangioma
- Malignancy: Lymphoma, neuroblastoma, parotid tumor, rhabdomyosarcoma

■ **Management**

- Determine most likely organism based on age, exposure, and examination

Bacterial Adenitis
- Empiric therapy
  - PO: Cephalexin or dicloxacillin (first line), or clindamycin, amoxicillin-clavulanate, cefuroxime, trimethoprim-sulfamethoxazole (TMP-SMX), ciprofloxacin, or linezolid
  - IV: oxacillin, cefazolin, clindamycin, ampicillin-sulbactam, TMP-SMX, or vancomycin
- Consider needle aspiration or incisional drainage if 1) not improved in 2 days; 2) suppuration

B. henselae
- Self-limited, resolves over 2 to 4 months
- Azithromycin for 5 days decreases lymph node volume more than placebo over first month
- Antibiotics with in vitro susceptibility include rifampin, macrolides, tetracyclines, TMP-SMX, quinolones, and aminoglycosides

NTM
- Standard therapy requires surgical resection of affected nodes
- Incisional drainage not recommended because it may lead to sinus tract drainage
- Medical management with clarithromycin, ethambutol, or rifampin rarely successful

M. tuberculosis
- Isoniazid, rifampin, and pyrazinamide ± ethambutol or streptomycin

■ **Complications**

- Compression of adjacent structures; draining sinus tract; extension to form deep neck abscess; bacteremia

Lower Respiratory Tract Infections

Samir S. Shah, MD

Bronchiolitis

- Acute viral lower respiratory tract infection

■ Epidemiology

- Peak occurrence in October through May
- 80% of infections occur in children younger than 2 years

■ Risk Factors

- Risk factors for severe illness during bronchiolitis: Chronic lung disease (CLD); cystic fibrosis; congenital heart disease (CHD); hematopoietic stem cell or organ transplantation; cellular immune deficits (e.g., 22q11.2 deletion)

■ Etiology

- Common: Respiratory syncytial virus (RSV; 70% of cases)
- Less common: Parainfluenza, influenza, adenovirus
- Rare: Human metapneumovirus, *Mycoplasma pneumoniae*, rhinovirus

■ Pathogenesis

- Virus induces
  - Desquamation of ciliated respiratory epithelial cells
  - Lymphocytic infiltration of peribronchial epithelial cells
- Intraluminal debris accumulates, mucosal edema worsens
- Resulting debris and edema obstruct small airways

■ History/Physical Examination

- Symptoms begin 2 to 8 days after exposure
- Initially low-grade fever, cough, and rhinorrhea
- Apnea can occur in those younger than 6 months
- Tachypnea, hypoxia, subcostal/intercostal retractions, rales, wheezing, rhonchi

■ Additional Studies

- Chest radiograph: Hyperinflation and patchy atelectasis
- Nasopharyngeal (NP) aspirate

- Rapid enzyme immunoassay for RSV and influenza: Sensitivity, 85%; specificity, 97%
- Fluorescent antibody: Antigens of RSV, influenza, parainfluenza, and adenovirus
- Viral culture

■ Differential Diagnosis

- Airway hypersensitivity to environmental irritants
- Gastroesophageal reflux with pulmonary aspiration
- Anatomic airway abnormality
- Cardiac disease with pulmonary edema
- Other causes of wheezing

■ Management

- Extent of bronchiolar necrosis and speed of regeneration influence recovery
- Usually self-limited: 3 to 7 days acute illness with slow recovery (2 weeks)
- 0.5% to 1% of patients require hospitalization; of these, 5% previously healthy and 20% high-risk require intubation

Relieving Airway Obstruction

- β-Agonists (nebulized albuterol)
  - Evidence on efficacy conflicting
  - Modest short-term improvement in clinical features *but* no impact on rate or duration of hospitalization
- Combined α- and β-agonists (racemic epinephrine)
  - In principle, α-agonist diminishes airway edema/mucous production and β-agonist relieves bronchospasm
  - No large trial but several small trials report conflicting results
- Corticosteroids (prednisone, dexamethasone)
  - In principle, reduce airway edema
  - No data supports use of *inhaled* steroids; poor data regarding use of *systemic* steroids
  - Steroids may benefit subgroups: 1) Previous wheezing, 2) severe illness, 3) treated early in illness

Antiviral Therapy and Prevention

- Therapy: Aerosolized ribavirin
  - Difficult and costly to deliver
  - Minimal clinical improvement in previously healthy children but early treatment benefits some high-risk children
- Prevention: Passive immunotherapy (antibody against RSV)
  - RSV intravenous immunoglobulin (RSV IVIG, RespiGam)
  - RSV-specific humanized monoclonal antibody (palivizumab, Synagis) (genetically engineered)

- No significant *therapeutic* benefit with either RSV IVIG or palivizumab
- Palivizumab monthly *prophylaxis* reduces RSV hospitalizations (from 8% to 2%) in children born prior to 32 weeks gestation

■ Complications

- Mortality: Less than 0.1% overall but 3% to 5% for those with CLD or CHD
- Long term: Asthma more likely but cause/effect unclear

Acute Pneumonia

■ Epidemiology

- Most common in children younger than 2 years
- Seven-valent pneumococcal vaccine (Prevnar) reduced *Streptococcus pneumoniae* bacteremic pneumonia by 90%

■ Risk Factors

- Anatomic abnormalities (e.g., cleft palate, tracheoesophageal fistula)
- Primary or acquired immune deficiency (e.g., Hyper IgE, HIV, chemotherapy)
- Physiologic abnormalities: 1) Swallowing dysfunction/severe gastroesophageal reflux; 2) dysmotile cilia syndromes; 3) altered mucous secretions (e.g., cystic fibrosis)

■ Etiology

- 30% to 40% bacterial; *S. pneumoniae* remains most common (Table 9-1)

■ Pathogenesis

- Three main mechanisms of infection
  - Transient or chronic impairment of normal airway defenses
  - Inhalation of large aerosol burden
  - Hematogenous seeding of the lung

■ History/Physical Examination

- Fever, cough, labored breathing, chest or abdominal pain, vomiting, decreased activity
- Tachypnea is the most reliable predictor of pneumonia in children: Sensitivity, 50% to 85%; Specificity, 70% to 95%
- Wheezing with pneumonia usually signifies viral or atypical cause
- Common findings:

▇ TABLE 9-1 Common Causes of Childhood Pneumonia by Age

Neonates	1–3 months	3 months–5 years	>5 years
Group B *Streptococcus*	Lower respiratory viruses[a]	Lower respiratory viruses	*Mycoplasma pneumoniae*
Gram-negative enteric bacilli	*Streptococcus pneumoniae*	*Streptococcus pneumoniae*	*Chlamydophila pneumoniae*
Cytomegalovirus	*Chlamydia trachomatis*	*Haemophilus influenzae*	*Streptococcus pneumoniae*
Listeria monocytogenes	*Bordetella pertussis*	*Mycoplasma pneumoniae*	Influenza viruses
Herpes simplex virus	*Staphylococcus aureus*		
Streptococcus pneumoniae	*Ureaplasma urealyticum*		

[a] Includes respiratory syncytial virus, adenovirus, parainfluenza viruses, and influenza viruses.

- General: Tachypnea, grunting, flaring, splinting, subcostal/intercostals retractions, dullness to percussion
- Auscultation: Rales, wheezing, tubular breath sounds, egophony, bronchophony, whispered pectoriloquy

▇ Additional Studies

- Chest radiograph (CXR) required for firm diagnosis
  - Consider CXR: 1) Young children, 2) uncertain/severe diagnosis, 3) failure of therapy, or 4) recurrent infections
- Diagnostic clues
  - Bacterial: Lobar/segmental consolidation or large pleural effusion
  - *Staphylococcus aureus*: Pneumatoceles (air-filled cavities from alveolar rupture)
  - Viral or atypical: Diffuse or bilateral interstitial pattern
  - 10% of *M. pneumoniae* infections lobar, 20% with small bilateral pleural effusions
- Blood cultures (uncomplicated pneumonia) positive in less than 2% of outpatients *but* 7% to 10% of hospitalized children
- Transthoracic needle aspiration: Microbiologic yield 70% with culture, polymerase chain reaction (PCR), and immunofluorescence
  - Consider if immunodeficient or worsening pneumonia of unclear cause
- NP cultures correlate poorly with cultures of lung tissue

- Diagnosis of specific agents (*, preferred initial test)
  - Viruses: Antigen detection* or viral culture of NP aspirate
  - *M. pneumoniae/C. pneumoniae*: PCR* of NP aspirate or serum antibodies
  - *C. trachomatis*: Direct fluorescent antibody* (DFA) or culture of NP/conjunctival swab
  - *Bordetella pertussis*: PCR*, DFA, or culture of NP aspirate
  - *Mycobacterium tuberculosis*: Intradermal skin test* (PPD), or acid-fast bacillus culture and smear of sputum, gastric aspirate, bronchoalveolar lavage, pleural biopsy, or pleural fluid

■ **Differential Diagnosis**

- Less common infectious causes
  - Fungal pneumonia in normal host (e.g., histoplasmosis)
  - Specific animal exposure (e.g., psittacosis, leptospirosis)
  - Unrecognized immunodeficiency (e.g., *Cryptococcus neoformans, Pneumocystis carinii*)
- Noninfectious conditions mimicking pneumonia: Foreign body aspiration, heart failure, malignancy, atelectasis, and sarcoidosis

■ **Management**

- Empiric therapy if bacterial cause suspected (Table 9-2); consider local susceptibility patterns
- Bacteriologic failure in drug-resistant *S. pneumoniae* pneumonia
  - Associated with second-generation cephalosporins and macrolides
  - *Not* associated with penicillin, ampicillin, or cefotaxime
- Typical duration of treatment: 10 to 14 days

■ TABLE 9-2 Empiric Therapy for Acute Pneumonia	
Age	**Empiric Treatment**
Neonate	First line: Ampicillin + gentamicin Alternative: Ampicillin + cefotaxime
1–3 months	First line: Amoxicillin or ampicillin [a] Alternative: Cefotaxime, vancomycin
3 months–5 years	First line: Amoxicillin or ampicillin Alternative: Cefotaxime, ceftriaxone, clindamycin, macrolide, vancomycin
>5 years	First line: Amoxicillin or ampicillin [b] Alternative: Cefotaxime, ceftriaxone, clindamycin, macrolide, levofloxacin, vancomycin

[a] Add macrolide if *C. trachomatis* or *B. pertussis* suspected.
[b] Consider adding macrolide or doxycycline or using fluoroquinolone as monotherapy to cover for atypical organisms.

■ **Complications**

• Pleural effusion, empyema, necrotizing pneumonia, abscess, sepsis

Pleural Effusion

• Fluid between the visceral and parietal pleura
  - Transudate: Nonpurulent effusion, usually nonpneumonic in origin
  - Exudate: Turbid, proteinaceous; usually infection, rarely malignancy
  - Empyema: Purulent; complicates bacterial pneumonia

■ **Epidemiology**

• Occurs in 0.5% of children with bacterial pneumonia
• Occurs in 13% to 36% with pneumonia who require hospitalization

■ **Risk Factors**

• Aspiration of gastrointestinal contents

■ **Etiology**

• Common: *S. pneumoniae*, *S. aureus*
• Less common: *M. tuberculosis*, group A *Streptococcus*, *Haemophilus influenzae*, *M. pneumoniae*, group B *Streptococcus* or enteric gram-negative rods (neonates), viruses (e.g., adenovirus, herpes simplex virus), *Blastomyces*, *Coccidioides*

■ **Pathogenesis**

• Pleural inflammation leads to effusion
• Exudative phase: Neutrophil migration into pleural space
• Fibrinopurulent phase: Fibrin deposition and loculation formation
• Organizing phase: Fibroblast formation produces inelastic membrane or "fibrinous peel"

■ **History**

• Suspect pleural effusion if: 1) Pleuritic chest pain, 2) fever more than 48 hours after starting treatment for pneumonia, 3) clinical deterioration during treatment of pneumonia

■ **Physical Examination**

• Dullness to lung percussion, diminished breath sounds over affected lung

■ **Additional Studies**

- Blood cultures positive in 10% to 25% of children with empyema
- CXR:
  - Upright: Blunted phrenic angle, air-fluid level, subpulmonic density
  - Decubitus: Layering differentiates free flowing from loculated
- Additional imaging: To assess for loculation (chest ultrasound or CT); to delineate anatomy (chest CT)
- Send pleural fluid studies (Box 9-1 and Table 9-3)
- Pleural fluid eosinophilia: Parasites, TB, fungi, or hypersensitivity diseases
- Consider pleural biopsy to detect tuberculous granulomas

■ BOX 9-1 Pleural Fluid Studies

Always
Cell count
Glucose
pH
LDH
Gram stain
Acid-fast stain
Cultures[a]

Sometimes
Mycoplasma PCR
Viral antigen immunofluorescence
Viral culture
Total protein
Amylase
Cholesterol
Cytology (to exclude malignancy)

[a] Aerobic and anaerobic, consider mycobacterial and fungal.

■ TABLE 9-3 Pleural Fluid Assessment

Test	Transudate	Exudate	Empyema
WBC (per mm³)	<1000	>5000	>10,000
Glucose (mg/dL)	>60	40–60	<40
pH	>7.3	7.2–7.3	<7.1
LDH (IU/L)	<200	200–1000	>1000
LDH (pleural/serum)	<0.6	>0.6	>0.6

■ **Differential Diagnosis**

- Capillary leak (e.g., sepsis)
- Increased hydrostatic pressure (e.g., congestive heart failure)
- Decreased oncotic pressure (e.g., hypoalbuminemia)
- Obstructed lymphatics (e.g., malignancy)
- Iatrogenic (e.g., misdirected nasogastric tube)

■ **Management**

- Start antimicrobial therapy based on probable pathogens and adjust based on blood/pleural fluid culture results
  - Empiric: Ampicillin-sulbactam or cefotaxime + oxacillin (vancomycin if methicillin-resistant *S. aureus* prevalent)
- Classify pleural effusions based on CXR results
  - Size on decubitus CXR
    - Small: Less than 10 mm
    - Moderate: 10 mm or more, but less than half of hemithorax
    - Large: Half of hemithorax or more
  - Character: Free flowing or loculated
- Surgical management options to prevent organizing phase and remove loculations/fibrinous peel
  - Thoracentesis (needle aspiration)
  - Tube thoracostomy (TT; chest tube) with or without fibrinolysis
  - Open decortication or video-assisted thoracoscopy (VATS) with decortication
- Initial surgical management based on size and character of effusion: 1) **Small:** No surgical management; 2) **Moderate:** Thoracentesis or TT; 3) **Large:** TT or VATS; 4) **Loculated:** Open decortication or VATS
- Subsequent management based on detection of empyema: 1) If initial thoracentesis reveals empyema, perform TT; 2) If inadequate drainage from TT, perform open decortication or VATS

■ **Complications**

- Restrictive lung defect; mortality highest in small infants and those with *S. aureus* infections

Pulmonary Lymphadenopathy

■ **Etiology**

- Any disease that affects the lung can cause pulmonary lymphadenopathy
- Some pathogens cause adenopathy out of proportion to parenchymal involvement (Box 9-2)

■ **BOX 9-2 Infectious Causes of Pulmonary Lymphadenopathy**

Bacterial
Mycobacterium tuberculosis
Nontuberculous mycobacteria
Mycoplasma pneumoniae
Bartonella henselae
Bordetella pertussis
Yersinia enterocolitica
Brucella spp.
Francisella tularensis

Fungal
Histoplasma capsulatum
Coccidioides immitis
Paracoccidioides brasiliensis
Blastomyces dermatitidis
Cryptococcus neoformans

Other
HIV
Epstein-Barr virus
Toxoplasma gondii

■ **Pathogenesis**

- Findings that suggest abnormal mediastinal lymph nodes: 1) Lymph nodes present where none usually seen; 2) size greater than 1.5 cm; 3) lymph node morphology reveals calcification, cavitation, caseation, or rim enhancement

■ **History**

- Findings from underlying cause or compression of adjacent structures. Inquire about:
  - Cough, wheezing, hemoptysis, dysphagia, hematemesis
  - Facial swelling, headaches, epistaxis, tinnitus
  - Hoarse voice, symptoms of spinal cord compression

■ **Physical Examination**

- Determine number, location, and size of lymph nodes outside the chest
- Findings from underlying cause or compression of adjacent structures. Adjacent structures include:
  - Trachea, bronchi, esophagus
  - Superior vena cava, lymphatic vessels
  - Recurrent laryngeal and phrenic nerves, sympathetic ganglia, ribs, vertebrae

■ Additional Studies

- CXR: Detects size and location of mass; detects calcifications; prompts further imaging (CT or MRI) to define anatomy and extent of disease
- Chest CT: Demonstrates calcium; better for anterior and middle mediastinal masses
- Chest MRI: Does not demonstrate calcium; better for posterior mediastinal masses (usually neurogenic origin)
- Tuberculin skin testing (PPD)
- Complete blood count findings (e.g., pancytopenia, eosinophilia) may suggest cause

■ Differential Diagnosis

- Chronic inflammation: Bronchiectasis, cystic fibrosis, lung abscess
- Malignancy: Hodgkin lymphoma, non-Hodgkin lymphoma, leukemia
- Other: Chronic granulomatous disease, Langerhans cell histiocytosis, sarcoidosis, Castleman disease

■ Management

- Lymph node biopsy if: 1) Other tests do not reveal cause; 2) size increases over 2 weeks or persists for more than 4 weeks; 3) malignancy is suspected

■ Complications

- Related to cause of mediastinal adenopathy

Cardiac Infections

Robert S. Baltimore, MD

Endocarditis

- Endocarditis: Infection on the endocardial surface of the heart including the heart valves
- Infections on the endothelial surface of blood vessels may act as "endocarditis"

■ Epidemiology

- Estimated incidence, 1.7 to 4 cases per 100,000 population per year in developed countries
- In children, mostly a complication of congenital heart disease (CHD)

■ Risk Factors

- CHD: Especially tetralogy of Fallot and ventricular septal defects
- Surgically repaired CHD using patches, grafts, or artificial valves
- Others: Mitral valve prolapse; atherosclerosis (adults); intravenous drug use; indwelling central vascular catheters; rheumatic heart disease (once common, now rare)

■ Etiology

- Bacteria: Viridans streptococci (most common at all ages); enterococci; *Staphylococcus aureus*; coagulase-negative staphylococci; hemolytic streptococci, groups A, B (in neonates and elderly), C, G, D *Streptococcus*; *Streptococcus pneumoniae*; gram-negative enteric rods (uncommon); HACEK organisms (*Haemophilus aphrophilus*, *Actinobacillus actinomycetemcomitans*, *Cardiobacterium hominis*, *Eikenella corrodens*, and *Kingella kingae*)
- Fungi: *Candida* species, *Aspergillus* species, *Cryptococcus neoformans*
- Others: *Coxiella burnetii* (Q fever), chlamydiae, culture-negative endocarditis

■ **Pathogenesis**

- Turbulent blood flow, regurgitant jet, or foreign body abrades endocardial surface
- Endocardial erosion allows platelet-fibrin thrombi to form
- Bacteria or fungi implant on thrombi resulting in vegetation formation
- Prosthetic heart material, cut surfaces, and foreign bodies allow bacteria to adhere

■ **History/Physical Examination (Box 10-1)**

- Key features: Change in heart murmur, new or worsening heart failure, peripheral septic emboli, or new neurologic findings

---

■ **BOX 10-1 Symptoms, Signs, and Laboratory Findings Associated with Infective Endocarditis in Children**

Symptoms
Fever
Malaise
Anorexia/weight loss
Heart failure
Arthralgia
Chest pain
Neurologic symptoms[a]
Gastrointestinal symptoms

Signs
Fever
Splenomegaly
Petechiae
Embolic phenomenon
New or changed murmur
Clubbing
Osler nodes
Roth spots
Janeway lesions
Splinter hemorrhages
Conjunctival hemorrhage

Laboratory Findings
Positive blood culture
Elevated ESR
Anemia
Positive rheumatoid factor
Hematuria

[a] Such as focal neurologic deficit and aseptic meningitis.

■ **Additional Studies (Box 10-1)**

- Echocardiography to visualize vegetations. Lesions as small as 2 mm can be seen
- Transesophageal echocardiography most sensitive for older children and for those with prosthetic valves but usually unnecessary in young children

■ **Differential Diagnosis**

- Best differentiated from other causes using the Duke criteria

■ **Management**

- Major indications for surgery in patients with endocarditis: 1) Persistent vegetation after systemic embolization; 2) increase in vegetation size after 4 weeks of antimicrobial therapy; 3) congestive heart failure not responding to medical treatment; 4) periannular extension of infection or abscess; 5) fungal endocarditis; 6) persistent bacteremia or emboli despite adequate antibiotic therapy; 7) unstable prosthesis
- Take multiple blood cultures (at least three) before antibiotic treatment
- Empiric antibiotics for the very ill but in subacute disease await results of blood cultures
- Antibiotic treatment with bactericidal drugs. Preferred regimens as follows:
  - Viridans streptococci, *S. bovis*: Penicillin or ceftriaxone with or without gentamicin
  - Enterococci: Penicillin (vancomycin if penicillin resistant) plus gentamicin
  - Methicillin-susceptible staphylococci: Nafcillin or oxacillin (vancomycin for methicillin-resistant *S. aureus*)
  - Staphylococci with prosthetic device or materials: Nafcillin, oxacillin, or cefazolin plus rifampin plus gentamicin

■ **Complications**

- Congestive heart failure, stroke, arrhythmia, metastatic infection, and mycotic aneurysms

Pericarditis

- Infection/inflammation of the pericardium surrounding the heart and proximal great vessels

■ **Epidemiology**

- Retrospective reviews: 2/1000 to 3/1000 admissions to children's hospitals

- In summer, usually enteroviruses. In winter, more likely influenza

■ Risk Factors/Etiology (Box 10-2)

- Viral pericarditis is more common in adults
- Bacterial pericarditis is more common in children younger than 2 years. Tuberculous pericarditis may occur in miliary disease.
- Risk factors: Immunocompromised state including HIV infection

■ Pathogenesis

- Seeding of the pericardium from 1) viral or bacterial bloodstream infection; 2) extension of myocarditis as myopericarditis; 3) direct extension from contiguous lung infection; 4) multifocal spread of bacteremia (other distant foci may exist); 5) postsurgical chest infection
- Inflammation causes fluid accumulation between visceral and parietal pericardium

■ History

- Precordial chest pain (difficult to elicit in the very young)
- Fever, irritability, and exercise intolerance
- Night sweats and hemoptysis in tuberculous pericarditis

■ BOX 10-2 Causes of Pericarditis

Viruses
Coxsackie B[a]
Coxsackie A
Echoviruses
Adenoviruses
Influenza

Bacteria
Staphylococcus aureus[a]
Haemophilus influenzae type b[a]
Neisseria meningitidis[a]
Mycobacterium tuberculosis

Others
Mycoplasma pneumoniae
Histoplasma capsulatum
Coccidioides immitis
Blastomyces dermatitidis

[a] Most common causes in North America.

■ Physical Examination

- May be accompanied by a viral rash
- Fever, cough, tachypnea, muffled heart sounds, friction rub
- Signs of chronic right-hearted congestive heart failure if constrictive pericarditis
- Pulsus paradoxus of more than 10 mm Hg suggests cardiac tamponade

■ Additional Studies

- Chest radiograph: Enlarged cardiac silhouette
- Two-dimensional and M-mode echocardiography: Detects pericardial fluid
- Pericardiocentesis: Diagnostic and therapeutic
  - Send for WBC and differential counts, glucose, protein, and cytology
  - Gram stain, acid-fast stain, and silver stain
  - Culture for viruses, bacteria (aerobic and anaerobic), fungi, and mycobacteria
- Viral cultures [and polymerase chain reaction (PCR) if available] from nasopharynx, throat, stool, and pericardial fluid
- Blood cultures for bacteria and fungi
- Serology (paired sera) for viruses, fungi, and mycoplasma
- Pericardial biopsy best for *Mycobacterium tuberculosis*
- ECG shows nonspecific ST-T wave changes (elevation or depression). There may be low-voltage QRS complexes, PR segment deviation (early), flat or inverted T waves (late)

■ Differential Diagnosis

- Noninfectious causes of pericarditis: Collagen vascular diseases; rheumatic fever; sarcoidosis; drugs (hydralazine, phenytoin); injury (myocardial infarction, chest trauma); metabolic (hypothyroidism, uremia); neoplastic; familial Mediterranean fever; Kawasaki disease

■ Management

- Bed rest, pain relief (NSAIDs), and cardiac monitoring
- Steroids not usually recommended *except* for acute tuberculous pericarditis
- Drainage of pericardial fluid (urgent need if tamponade developing)
- Empiric antibiotics if bacterial pericarditis is suspected (oxacillin or nafcillin plus a third-generation cephalosporin such as ceftriaxone). For nosocomially-acquired infections, use vancomycin and ceftazidime with or without an aminoglycoside.
- Tuberculous pericarditis treated as for extrapulmonary tuberculosis

■ **Complications**

- Constrictive pericarditis may occur with any etiology; requires pericardiectomy

Myocarditis

- Inflammatory condition involving the myocardium; pericardium and endocardium sometimes involved. Dilated cardiomyopathy is a manifestation of chronic myocarditis

■ **Epidemiology/Risk Factors**

- Myocarditis follows 34.6 per 1000 coxsackie virus infections
- Certain agents vary geographically: For example, Chagas disease (South America) and Lyme disease (East and West Coast, Northern Midwest in United States)
- Risk factors include young age (particularly newborns) due to lack of protective antibody; immunocompromised including HIV

■ **Etiology**

- Common: Enteroviruses (particularly coxsackie viruses B3 and B4), adenoviruses
  - Formerly "idiopathic" cases probably due to coxsackie virus based on molecular probes
- Less common: Influenza A and B viruses, CMV, HIV, and Lyme disease
- Rare: Acute rheumatic fever, measles, varicella, *Corynebacterium diphtheriae* (toxin mediated), *Neisseria meningitidis, S. aureus, Haemophilus influenzae* type b

■ **Pathogenesis**

- Myocardium damaged by direct myocyte invasion followed by immune-mediated inflammation. Myocardial injury impairs contractility

■ **History/Physical Examination**

- Palpitations, fatigue, exercise intolerance, tachypnea, and chest pain (variable)
- Sometimes asymptomatic. Some viral infections cause associated hepatitis or encephalitis
- Arrhythmia or signs of congestive heart failure may be present: Tachycardia, tachypnea, elevated jugular venous pulses, S_3 gallop, cardiomegaly, crackles or hypoxia from pulmonary edema, hepatic enlargement, and pedal edema
- In infants may mimic sepsis or congenital heart disease

■ Additional Studies

- Cultures: viral (nasopharynx, throat, urine, stool, CSF); bacterial (blood, CSF, pericardial)
- Chest radiograph: Cardiac enlargement and pulmonary edema
- Endomyocardial biopsy for culture, histopathology, and PCR for viruses and *Borrelia burgdorferi*
  - PCR detects viral genome weeks to months after infection
- Use Dallas Criteria for histopathologic analysis of stage of inflammation in biopsy
- Elevated WBC, ESR, creatine phosphokinase (MB fraction), and cardiac troponin T
- ECG: Prolonged PR interval, low-voltage QRS (less than 5 mm), premature atrial and ventricular complexes, ST- and T-wave abnormalities, heart block, rhythm abnormalities
- Echocardiography: Decreased myocardial function (ejection fraction), detects pericarditis, endocarditis, and congenital heart disease
- Serology for *B. burgdorferi*, enteroviruses, *Trypanosoma cruzi*

■ Differential Diagnosis

- Pericarditis, endocarditis, myocardial infarction, congenital heart disease
- Noninfectious myocarditis associated with collagen vascular diseases, thyrotoxicosis, drugs (e.g., alcohol, cocaine), reactions to stinging insects, rheumatic fever, sarcoid, and Kawasaki disease

■ Management

- Supportive care including antiarrhythmics and inotropes
- Steroids probably not indicated in early acute disease but may benefit those with ongoing inflammation. Immunosuppressives unproven benefit
- IVIG beneficial in some research studies
- Lyme disease and other bacterial infections: Treat as for severe disseminated infection due to the specific agent. No proven role for antiviral agents (herpes may be an exception)

■ Complications

- Arrhythmia, congestive heart failure, dilated cardiomyopathy (from chronic inflammation)
- Progressive disease may require cardiac transplantation

11 Gastrointestinal Tract Infections

Petar Mamula, MD, Raman Sreedharan, MD, MRCPCH, and Kurt A. Brown, MD

Gastroenteritis

- Acute diarrhea: Abrupt increase of fluid content in stool (more than 10 mL/kg/d). Frequency of bowel movements ranges from 1 to 20 or more times per day
- Chronic diarrhea: Diarrhea lasting more than 14 days

■ Epidemiology/Risk Factors

- Worldwide: 1 billion episodes; 3 million to 5 million deaths annually in children
- US: 1 to 2 episodes per year in children younger than 5 years; 300 to 400 deaths per year
- Child care/nosocomial outbreaks (enteric viruses, *Giardia lamblia*); travel to developing country (*Campylobacter, Shigella,* or *Salmonella* spp., enterotoxigenic *Escherichia coli*); antibiotic-associated (*Clostridium difficile*); seafood (*Vibrio* spp., *Plesiomonas shigelloides*)

■ Etiology (Acute Infectious Diarrhea)

- **Viruses:** Rotavirus, calicivirus, astrovirus, enteric adenovirus (types 40 and 41)
- **Bacteria:**
  - Common: *Campylobacter jejuni, Shigella* spp., *Salmonella* spp., *E. coli*
  - Less common: *Yersinia enterocolitica, Bacillus cereus, C. difficile*
  - Rare: *Vibrio* spp., *Staphylococcus aureus, Clostridium perfringens, P. shigelloides, Aeromonas hydrophila*
- **Other:** See next section for discussion of intestinal parasites. Immunocompromised hosts may be infected with cytomegalovirus (CMV), herpes simplex virus (HSV), *Cryptosporidium ovale*.

■ Pathogenesis

- Many pathogens use more than one mechanism

- Noninflammatory: Affects proximal small bowel by enterotoxin adherence. Causes watery diarrhea. Examples: *Vibrio cholerae, Y. enterocolitica*
- Inflammatory: Invade GI tract epithelium. May cause dysentery. Examples: *Salmonella* and *Shigella* spp.

■ History

- Food- or water-borne illness
  - Incubation: Less than 6 hours (preformed toxin: *S. aureus, B. cereus*); 8 to 16 hours (*C. perfringens, B. cereus*); 16 to 96 hours (*Shigella, Salmonella, Vibrio* spp., invasive *E. coli, C. jejuni, Y. enterocolitica,* caliciviruses)
- Determine duration of illness, stooling pattern (frequency, volume, blood/mucus), travel and ingestion history (see "Epidemiology/Risk Factors"), hydration status
- Other symptoms: Fever, emesis, abdominal pain, rash, tenesmus

■ Physical Examination

- Signs of dehydration: Absence of tears, dry mucous membranes, decreased skin turgor, prolonged capillary refill, cool peripheral skin temperature, diminished pulse volume and elevated rate, and normal or low blood pressure
- Gastrointestinal: Tenderness, abdominal distention or mass, bowel sounds, rectal examination with hemoccult testing

■ Additional Studies

- Stool examination for blood and leukocytes
  - Positive fecal leukocyte examination indicates presence of an invasive or cytotoxin-producing organism such as *Shigella* spp., *Salmonella enteritidis, C. jejuni,* invasive *E. coli, C. difficile, Y. enterocolitica, Vibrio parahaemolyticus,* or *Aeromonas*
- Stool culture for bacteria (see Chapter 1)
- Consider stool antigen testing for rotavirus, adenovirus, *Giardia,* and *Cryptosporidium* (also see "Intestinal Parasites")

■ Differential Diagnosis

- Anatomic (e.g., Hirschsprung enterocolitis, short bowel syndrome, malrotation)
- Malabsorption (e.g., celiac disease, fructose intolerance, sucrase or lactase deficiency, Shwachman disease, glucose-galactose transport defect)
- Neoplasms (e.g., neuroblastoma, pheochromocytoma)
- Poisoning (e.g., heavy metals, mushrooms, scombroid)
- Endocrinopathy (e.g., thyrotoxicosis, Addison disease)
- Food allergy (e.g., cow milk or soy protein)

■ TABLE 11-1 Antimicrobial Therapy for Bacterial Enteropathogens

Bacteria	Indication	Antibiotic
Aeromonas spp.	Prolonged disease	TMP-SMX, ciprofloxacin
Campylobacter jejuni	Severe or systemic infection, immunodeficiency	Azithromycin, fluoroquinolones, erythromycin
Clostridium difficile	Symptomatic, not improving	Metronidazole (PO/IV) or oral vancomycin or cholestyramine
Escherichia coli	Severe or systemic infection	TMP-SMX, fluoroquinolones[a]
Salmonella spp.	Age <3 months, immunodeficiency, dissemination	Ampicillin, cefotaxime, ciprofloxacin, azithromycin
Shigella spp.	Dysentery	Ceftriaxone, azithromycin, fluoroquinolones, TMP-SMX
Vibrio cholerae	Treatment decreases illness duration	Ciprofloxacin, TMP-SMX, tetracyclines
Yersinia enterocolitica	Sepsis, immunodeficiency	Cefotaxime, TMP- SMX, fluoroquinolones

[a] Antibiotic management of *E. coli* 0157:H7 may increase risk of hemolytic-uremic syndrome.

- Miscellaneous (e.g., inflammatory bowel disease, vasculitis, laxative abuse)

■ Management
- Fluid and electrolyte replacement; precautions to prevent spread of enteropathogen; specific therapy if indicated (Table 11-1)

■ Complications
- Extraintestinal manifestations:
  - Erythema nodosum (*Campylobacter, Salmonella, Y. enterocolitica*)
  - Hemolytic-uremic syndrome (*E. coli, Shigella dysenteriae, Salmonella typhi, C. jejuni*)
  - Reactive arthritis (*C. difficile, C. jejuni, S. dysenteriae, S. enteritidis, C. ovale, Y. enterocolitica*)
  - Seizures (*S. dysenteriae*)

Intestinal Parasites

■ Epidemiology/Etiology
See Table 11-2.

■ **TABLE 11-2 Parasitic Intestinal Infections**

Parasite	Geographic Distribution	Treatment	Alternative Therapy
Stomach			
Anisakis sp.	Scandinavia, Holland, Japan, Pacific Coast of South America	Endoscopic or surgical larvae removal	—
Small Intestine			
Giardia lamblia	Prevalence highest in developing world (up to 30%)	Metronidazole (5 mg/kg TID × 3 d)	Tinidazole, mepacrine, furazolidone, paromomycin, quinacrine
Blastocystis hominis	Worldwide	Metronidazole (20–35 mg/kg divided TID × 10 d)	Furazolidone, tinidazole
Cryptosporidium parvum	Countries with high AIDS prevalence	Nitazoxanide (100–200 mg BID) (therapy only needed for patients with AIDS)	Azithromycin + paromomycin
Isospora belli	S. America, Africa, SE Asia	Trimethoprim (5 mg/kg)-sulfamethoxazole (25 mg/kg) BID × 7–10 d	Pyrimethamine (50–75 mg/day) + folinic acid
Cyclospora cayetanensis	Developing countries	Same as for *Isospora belli*	—
Strongyloides stercoralis	Tropics, eastern Europe, Australia, southern US	Albendazole (400 mg BID × 3 d), ivermectin (200 ìg/kg/d × 1–2 d)	Thiabendazole (25 mg/kg BID × 2–3 d)
Trichinella spiralis	Worldwide in communities consuming pork meat	Mebendazole (200 mg TID × 3 d, followed by 400 mg TID × 10 d)	—
Ascaris lumbricoides (roundworm)	Prevalence highest in developing world	Albendazole (200–400 mg single dose) or mebendazole (500 mg single dose)	Levamisole (5 mg/kg single dose), piperazine citrate, pyrantel pamoate
Ankylostoma duodenale (hookworm)	Africa, Asia, Australia, southern Europe	Mebendazole (100 mg BID × 3 d)	Albendazole (400 mg single dose)
Necator americanus (hookworm)	Central and South America, SE Asia, Pacific	Mebendazole (100 mg BID × 3 d)	Albendazole (400 mg single dose)
Taenia saginata	Worldwide, more in Central Africa	Praziquantel (5–10 mg/kg single dose)	Niclosamide (50 mg/kg single dose)

■ **Risk Factors**

- Immunocompromised host; immigration from or travel to endemic areas
- Day care attendance; contact with infected animals
- Contaminated food or water (including swimming pools)

■ **Pathogenesis**

- Transmission almost exclusively by fecal-oral route
- Involvement may vary from asymptomatic carriage to invasive infection

■ **History/Physical Examination**

- Travel and dietary history
- Abdominal pain, diarrhea, tenesmus, bloating, flatulence
- Fever, emesis, anorexia
- Wheezing (*Strongyloides stercoralis, Ascaris lumbricoides*)
- Muscle pain or skin rash (*Trichinella spiralis*)
- Pruritis ani (often nocturnal) (*Enterobius vermicularis*)
- Local skin reaction at the site of larvae penetration (*S. stercoralis, Ankylostoma duodenale*)
- Failure to thrive and growth impairment with chronic infections
- Evaluate for dehydration, abdominal obstruction or mass

■ **Additional Studies**

- Stool for ova and parasites (see Chapter 1): Several not found on standard ova and parasite testing (*Cryptosporidium parvum, Cyclospora cayetanensis,* and *Microsporidia* species)
- Duodenal aspirate (during endoscopy, or swallowed string test)
- Tape test (*E. vermicularis*)
- Mucosal biopsy (*G. lamblia, S. stercoralis, C. parvum, Entamoeba histolytica*)
- Enzyme-linked immunosorbent assay (ELISA) for giardiasis, amebiasis, cryptosporidiosis
- Serology for helmintic infections (*S. stercoralis,* trichinosis)
- Serum eosinophilia
- Muscle biopsy (*T. spiralis*)

■ **Management**

See Table 11-2.

■ **Complications**

- Hepatic abscess (amebiasis)
- Seizures (*Taenia solium*)
- Pneumonitis, myocarditis, encephalitis (*T. spiralis*)

- Intestinal and biliary obstruction, intussusception (*A. lumbricoides*)
- Iron deficiency anemia (*A. duodenale*)
- Megaloblastic anemia (*Diphyllobothrium latum*)
- Rectal prolapse (*Trichuris trichiura*)

Hepatitis

- Hepatitis: Clinical or biochemical evidence of hepatic dysfunction
- Classification: Acute (less than 6 months) or chronic (more than 6 months)

■ Epidemiology

- Schistosomiasis is most common cause worldwide (more than 200 million per year)
- Hepatitis B: 0.1% incidence in North America
- Hepatitis C: Prevalence is 1.8% of the general population in the United States, seroprevalence in children 0 to 12 years old is 0.2%

■ Risk Factors

- Poor hygiene, contaminated water (hepatitis A and E, parasites)
- Intravenous drug use; sex with an infected person; blood transfusion; hemodialysis; medical personnel exposed to blood; body piercing and tattooing (hepatitis B and C, HIV)
- Maternal-fetal transmission (hepatitis B and C, HIV)

■ Etiology/Pathogenesis (Box 11-1)

- Cellular hepatocyte damage may occur due to direct cytopathic effect or, more commonly, due to immune-mediated injury

■ History/Physical Examination

- Fever, fatigue, anorexia
- Jaundice, scleral icterus, abdominal pain, pruritus, diarrhea, dark urine
- Hepatomegaly (often painful), splenomegaly (with viruses)
- Rash (e.g., syphilis, Lyme disease, hepatitis B)

■ Additional Studies

- Elevated alanine aminotransferase (ALT) or aspartate aminotransferase (AST)
- ALT (mainly present in the liver) is more specific for liver disease than AST
- Elevated bilirubin, alkaline phosphatase, and γ-glutamyltransferase (GGT) suggest cholestasis
- Liver synthetic function: Serum albumin level, prothrombin time (PT) and partial thromboplastin time (PTT)

◼ **BOX 11-1 Causes of Infectious Hepatitis by Type of Organism**

Virus
Hepatitis virus A, B, C, D, E, G
Cytomegalovirus
Epstein-Barr virus
Herpes simplex virus
Adenovirus
Enterovirus
Coxsackie virus
HIV
Echovirus
Reovirus

Bacteria
Salmonella typhi (typhoid fever)
Brucella melitensis (brucellosis)
Bartonella henselae (cat-scratch)
Borrelia burgdorferi (Lyme disease)
Leptospira interrogans (leptospirosis)
Rickettsia rickettsii
Coxiella burnetii (Q fever)
Treponema pallidus (syphilis)

Parasite
Entamoeba histolytica (amebiasis)
Plasmodium spp. (malaria)
Ascaris lumbricoides
Echinococcus granulosus
Schistosoma species
Clonorchis sinensis (liver fluke)
Fasciola hepatica
Leishmania donovani
Toxocara canis

Fungi
Candida species
Histoplasma capsulatum
Aspergillus species
Cryptococcus neoformans
Coccidioides immitis
Penicillium marneffei
Trichosporon cutaneum

- Serologic tests for hepatitis viruses (Table 11-3)
- Abdominal ultrasound of the liver, biliary tree, and spleen to diagnose anatomic abnormalities
- Percutaneous liver biopsy may be required for diagnosis

■ TABLE 11-3 Interpretation of Serologic Tests in Hepatitis A, B, C, D, and E

Virus	Test	Acute Disease	Chronic Disease	Complete Recovery
Hepatitis A	HA IgM	+	N/A	−
	HA IgG	+	N/A	+
Hepatitis B	HBsAg	+	+	−
	HBsAb	−	−	+
	HBcAb	+ (IgM)	+ (IgG)	+ (IgG)
Hepatitis C	HCV PCR	+	+	−
	HCV Ab	+	+	+
Hepatitis D	HDV Ag	+	+	−
	HDV IgM	+	−	−
	HDV IgG	−	+	−
Hepatitis E	HE Ag	+	N/A	−
	HE IgM	+	N/A	−
	HDV PCR	+	N/A	−

■ **Differential Diagnosis**

- Cholecystitis, drug/toxin-induced, autoimmune hepatitis, Wilson disease, α_1-antitrypsin deficiency, inborn metabolic errors, sclerosing cholangitis, hepatic malignancy, vascular disorders (e.g., Budd-Chiari), others (Crohn)

■ **Management**

- Antibiotic treatment of bacterial, parasitic, and fungal hepatitis depends on the individual organism and severity of disease
- Most viral hepatitides are self-limited (e.g., CMV, Epstein-Barr, hepatitis A and E)
- Hepatitis B and C may progress to chronic hepatitis and require specific therapy to minimize complications
  - Hepatitis B: Subcutaneous interferon-α (three times a week for 4 to 6 months), or oral lamivudine
  - Hepatitis C: Pegylated interferon, and oral ribavirin

■ **Complications**

- Chronic hepatitis B and C: Cirrhosis, portal hypertension, and hepatocellular carcinoma (1.5 cases per 100 patients with cirrhosis). Fulminant hepatitis in 5% with hepatitis B and D coinfection
- Ascariasis, schistosomiasis, fascioliasis: Abscess or biliary obstruction
- Echinococcosis: Hydatid cyst formation, anaphylaxis with cyst rupture

Peritonitis

- Primary spontaneous bacterial peritonitis (SBP): Pathogenic bacteria in peritoneal fluid *without* an identified intra-abdominal source of infection
- Secondary bacterial peritonitis: Peritoneal infection *secondary* to an abdominal source, such as perforation of an abdominal viscus

■ Epidemiology/Risk Factors

- Risk factors: Appendicitis; chronic renal failure (occurs in up to 17% of patients with nephrotic syndrome); liver failure; peritoneal dialysis; ventriculoperitoneal (VP) shunt
- Also occurs in 2% to 17% of processes that perforate intestine (e.g., trauma, necrotizing enterocolitis, volvulus)

■ Etiology

- Common: *Streptococcus pneumoniae* (previously healthy children), S. *aureus* (dialysis catheters, VP shunts), gram-negative enteric bacilli (cirrhosis), coagulase-negative staphylococci (VP shunts)
- Less common: *Candida* spp., *Neisseria meningitidis*, *Haemophilus influenzae* type b (unimmunized)

■ Pathogenesis

- Primary SBP: Hematogenous or lymphatic spread to peritoneum
- Secondary bacterial peritonitis: Intestinal perforation

■ History/Physical Examination

- 10% of patients are entirely asymptomatic
- Acute febrile illness (50% to 80%), generalized abdominal pain
- Rebound tenderness, decreased bowel sounds, diarrhea, hypotension

■ Additional Studies

Paracentesis:
- Free air, blood, or bile suggest intestinal perforation
- WBCs in peritoneal fluid greater than 250/mm^3 support the diagnosis of peritonitis (often more than 3000/mm^3)
- In secondary bacterial peritonitis, ascitic fluid analysis usually reveals: Total protein greater than 1 g/L; lactate greater than 25 mg/dL; Glucose less than 50 mg/dL

■ *Blood cultures:*

- Blood cultures positive in 75% of primary SBP and occasionally with secondary bacterial peritonitis

■ Differential Diagnosis

- Other infections may mimic peritonitis: Mesenteric adenitis, gastroenteritis, streptococcal pharyngitis, lower lobe pneumonia, urinary tract infection

■ Management

- Empiric therapy: Cefotaxime or ceftriaxone
  - Add vancomycin for life-threatening or VP shunt–related infections
  - Add aminoglycoside for secondary bacterial peritonitis
  - Alternative regimens: Ampicillin-sulbactam, ticarillin-clavulanate, piperacillin-tazobactam, or carbapenem antibiotics
  - Repeat paracentesis may be indicated after 48 hours to ensure waning WBC count. If WBC count remains elevated or organisms continue to be cultured, suspect antibiotic-resistant organisms or secondary bacterial peritonitis.
- Secondary bacterial peritonitis: Surgical intervention to resolve underlying cause of abdominal infection

■ Complications

- Mortality: 30% to 40%; probability of primary SBP recurrence at one year is 70%; respiratory compromise may occur due to secondary to diaphragmatic spasm and abdominal rigidity

Cholangitis

- Pathologic biliary system inflammation

■ Epidemiology/Risk Factors

- Any disease with poor bile flow leading to biliary stasis. Especially:
  - Biliary drainage via a Roux-en-Y limb that approximates the small intestine to the porta hepatis (Kasai procedure for biliary atresia)
  - Liver transplantation (occurs in 10% of transplants, usually in first 2 months)
  - Intrahepatic cholestatic liver diseases (e.g., Alagille syndrome)

■ Etiology

- Common: *E. coli*, *Klebsiella* spp., *Enterococcus*, anaerobes (10% to 30% of cases)

- Less common: *Enterobacter* spp., *Pseudomonas aeruginosa*
- Rare: Other gram-negative bacilli, *Cryptococcus* (HIV), *Cryptosporidium*

■ Pathogenesis

- Bile is typically sterile
- Biliary infection due to either ascending infection from gut lumen or hematogenous spread from portal venous circulation during bacteremia

■ History/Physical Examination

- History of cholestatic liver disease
- Charcot triad (fever/chills, right upper quadrant pain, jaundice) in more than 50%

■ Additional Studies

- Elevated transaminases or bilirubin from baseline
- Alkaline phosphatase or GGT commonly are elevated
- Blood cultures positive in approximately 50%
- Bile or hepatic (via biopsy) cultures usually positive

■ Differential Diagnosis

- Esophagitis, gastritis, gastroesophageal reflux, cholecystitis, pancreatitis, appendicitis, Fitz-Hugh-Curtis syndrome, pneumonia

■ Management

- Empiric antibiotics: Ampicillin-sulbactam with or without aminoglycoside or cefotaxime plus metronidazole
  - Alternative regimens: Ticarcillin-clavulanate; carbapenems; ciprofloxacin plus metronidazole.
- If fever persists longer than 72 hours, consider percutaneous liver biopsy with culture
- No consistently demonstrated benefit of antibiotic prophylaxis for recurrences

■ Complications

- Pyogenic liver abscess; recurrent cholangitis

Genitourinary Tract Infections

Ron Keren, MD, MPH and David Rubin, MD, MSCE

Urinary Tract Infection

- Urinary tract infection (UTI): Infection of the bladder (cystitis, lower tract) or kidneys (pyelonephritis, upper tract)

■ Epidemiology

- Prevalence in febrile children without fever source: Ages 2 to 24 months = 5%
  - Gender is an important variable in those older than 3 months (e.g., prevalence at ages 12 to 24 months: boys = 1.9%; girls = 8.1%)

■ Risk Factors/ Etiology (Box 12-1)

- White race (in school-aged girls); uncircumcised phallus (5 to 20 times increased risk); sexually active female; male sex (younger than 3 months); female sex (older than 3 months); indwelling urinary catheter; vesicoureteral reflux (VUR)

■ Pathogenesis

- GI bacteria colonize periurethral mucosa (mediated by host and bacterial adhesion factors) and then ascend to bladder and kidneys
- VUR (present in 30% to 50% with UTI) increases risk of pyelonephritis

■ History/Physical Examination

- Infants: Fever, irritability, decreased feeding/activity, vomiting, jaundice (neonates)
- Pre–school age: Fever, abdominal pain, enuresis, foul-smelling urine
- School age: Dysuria, frequency, urgency, hesitancy, hematuria, back/abdominal pain
- **Fever** in a child with a positive urine culture reliably identifies pyelonephritis (sensitivity = 84%, specificity = 92%)
- **Exam findings** do *not* reliably distinguish cystitis from pyelonephritis. Up to 25% of children without signs/symptoms

■ BOX 12-1 Causes of Urinary Tract Infection

Common
E. coli[a]
Proteus spp.[b]
Klebsiella spp.
P. aeruginosa
Enterococcus spp.
S. saprophyticus

Less Common
Group B streptococci
Salmonella spp.
Shigella spp.
Campylobacter spp.

Rare
H. influenzae type b
Anaerobes
Fungi
M. tuberculosis
Protozoa
Adenovirus

[a] Accounts for 70% to 90% of UTIs.
[b] Usually in boys older than 1 year.

of pyelonephritis have bacteria isolated from kidneys by ureteral catheterization.
• Meatal erythema or abnormalities, costovertebral angle or suprapubic tenderness

■ Additional Studies (Table 12-1)

• Urine dipstick positive (dipstick positive if ≥ trace leukocyte esterase or positive nitrite): Sensitivity = 80%; specificity = 97%
• Urine dipstick positive or 5 or more bacteria per high-powered field by microscopy: Sensitivity = 85%; specificity = 87%

■ Differential Diagnosis

• Urethritis, vaginitis, cervicitis, prostatitis, foreign body, nephrolithiasis, renal abscess, vaginovesical fistula, enterovesical fistula

■ Management

• Well-appearing children with a urinalysis suspicious for UTI require antibiotics while awaiting confirmatory culture results;

■ **TABLE 12-1 Interpretation of the Urine Culture**

Collection Method	Colony Count[a]	Probability of Infection
Suprapubic aspirate	Any number[b]	>99%
Transurethral catheterization	>100,000	95%
	10,000–100,000	Probable
	1000–10,000	Possible (repeat)
	<1000	Unlikely
Clean void	3 Specimens >100,000	95%
	1 Specimen >100,000	80%
	10,000–100,000	Possible (repeat)
	<10,000	Unlikely

[a] Colony count of pure culture.
[b] If gram-negative bacilli.
Adapted from American Academy of Pediatrics. Practice parameter: the diagnosis, treatment, and evaluation of the initial urinary tract infection in febrile infants and young children. *Pediatrics* 1999;103:843–852.

some evidence that these patients can be treated safely as out-patients with *oral* antibiotics
- Children 2 to 24 months of age with suspected UTI assessed as toxic, dehydrated, or unable to retain oral intake require *parenteral* antibiotics and fluids
- Empiric antibiotic therapy:
  - IV: Ampicillin plus gentamicin (combined) or cefotaxime (monotherapy)
  - PO: Ceftibuten, TMP-SMX, cephalexin, or amoxicillin-clavulanate
- Duration of therapy: 10 to 14 days
- For children 2 to 24 months with UTI, the AAP recommends 1) renal ultrasound to identify congenital or acquired urinary tract abnormalities (e.g., dysplasia, hydronephrosis); 2) voiding cystourethrogram (VCUG) to identify VUR, and, in boys, posterior urethral valves
- Renal cortical scintigraphy 99mTechnitium-dimercaptosuccinic acid (DMSA) scan identifies acute pyelonephritis and renal scarring. Not routinely required

■ **Complications**
- Bacteremia (18% risk if 1 to 3 months old; but rare if older than 1 year); perinephric abscess or stones; renal scarring causing hypertension and end-stage renal disease

Renal Abscess (Intrarenal and Perinephric)

- Intrarenal abscess: Collection of purulent material within the kidney
- Perinephric abscess: Abscess outside the kidney but within the renal fascia

■ Epidemiology

- Uncommon but exact incidence unknown; affects all age groups; no gender preference

■ Risk Factors

- Urinary tract: Infection, VUR, obstruction, neurogenic bladder, nephrolithiasis, tumor, polycystic kidney disease, peritoneal dialysis
- Other conditions: Bacteremia; abdominal or urinary tract surgery; immunodeficiency; renal trauma; diabetes mellitus

■ Etiology

- Common: Enterobacteriaceae (primarily *Escherichia coli*); *Staphylococcus aureus*
- Less common: *Pseudomonas* spp.; *Enterococcus* spp.; coagulase-negative staphylococci (prosthetic device related); *Streptococcus* spp.; *Candida* spp.
- Rare: *Actinomyces*; anaerobic organisms; *Mycobacterium tuberculosis*

■ Pathogenesis

- Intrarenal abscess: Usually hematogenous spread (*Staphylococcus aureus*); occasionally complication of ascending UTI (Enterobacteriaceae)
- Perinephric abscess: Usually complication of ascending UTI or direct extension of intrarenal abscess; occasionally hematogenous spread

■ History

- One to three weeks of malaise, lethargy, weight loss, nausea, vomiting, fever, and costovertebral angle tenderness or referred to back, abdomen or hip, UTI symptoms (if antecedent UTI)
- Consider abscess if: 1) Failed UTI treatment; 2) fever without source after urinary or abdominal surgery; and 3) fever and urinary tract obstruction

■ Physical Examination

- Palpable renal mass (5% of cases, mostly infants), scoliosis with splinting of affected side, pain on bending to contralateral side

■ Additional Studies

- ESR and peripheral WBC count: Elevated in 90%
- Urinalysis: Microscopic pyuria
- Cultures: Blood (positive in 35% of cases); urine (positive in 50% of cases)
- Gram stain and culture abscess fluid at time of aspiration or drainage (aerobic and anaerobic bacteria, fungi, and mycobacteria)
- Imaging studies: Ultrasound with Doppler, MRI, CT, renal cortical scintigraphy

■ Differential Diagnosis

- Pyelonephritis, hydronephrosis, renal dysplasia, renal tumor, renal vein thrombosis

■ Management

- Intravenous antibiotics active against Enterobacteriaceae and *S. aureus* (oxacillin or nafcillin and aminoglycoside or cefotaxime)
- Add antibiotic with anaerobic activity in patients with urinary obstruction or anaerobic infection elsewhere
- Expect clinical response (defervescence, decreased pain) to antibiotic with 2 to 3 days
- If not responding:
  - Ultrasound-guided percutaneous aspiration for diagnosis, culture, and cytology, with or without catheter drain placed
  - Open surgical drainage if percutaneous aspiration not successful
  - Nephrectomy if abscess is massive and kidney function unlikely to be preserved

■ Complications

- Loss of renal function; extension within kidney or perinephric space; rupture into abdominal or pulmonary space; hematogenous spread to other sites

Pelvic Inflammatory Disease and Cervicitis

- Pelvic inflammatory disease (PID): Ascending spread of microorganisms up the genitourinary tract. Distinguish PID from uncomplicated cervicitis (vaginal discharge and cervical findings without abdominal pain)

■ Epidemiology/Risk Factors

- 20% of all cases occur in adolescents; 1 in 8–10 sexually active are affected

- Increased risk: Young age, multiple partners, history of STD, intrauterine device use
- Decreased risk: Barrier contraceptive, vaginal spermicide

■ Etiology

- Acute infection: *Neisseria gonorrhoeae, Chlamydia trachomatis*
- Subacute or recurrent infection:
  - Anaerobes: *Bacteroides* spp., *Clostridium* spp., *Peptostreptococcus, Actinomyces*
  - Aerobes: *E. coli, Haemophilus influenzae, Streptococcus* spp.

■ History/Physical Examination

- Clinical diagnosis complicated by high rate of asymptomatic infection
- Signs and symptoms include: lower abdominal pain, acute onset (95%), adnexal tenderness (90%), vaginal discharge (55%), irregular menstrual bleeding (35%), fever (35%), urethritis (20%), vomiting (10%), proctitis (10%)
- Often occurs within 7 days of menses (unlike ectopic pregnancy)

Criteria for Diagnosis of PID

- Minimal criteria (60% of all cases): Lower abdominal tenderness, adnexal tenderness, and cervical motion tenderness
- Supportive criteria: Fever; vaginal discharge; elevated CRP or ESR; laboratory documented infection with *N. gonorrhoeae* or *C. trachomatis*
- Definitive criteria: Histopathologic evidence by endometrial biopsy; radiologic imaging revealing fluid-filled and thickened fallopian tubes; laparoscopic diagnosis

■ Additional Studies

- Cervical culture for *N. gonorrhoeae* and *C. trachomatis*
- Nucleic acid amplification (rapid detection with PCR/LCR) techniques replacing culture as tests of choice
- Consider testing for other STDs including HIV and syphilis
- Exclude pregnancy (including ectopic)
- Abdominal/pelvic ultrasound: Fluid-filled/thick fallopian tubes; tubo-ovarian abscess

■ Differential Diagnosis

- Gynecologic causes: Pregnancy (including ectopic), ovarian cyst, ovarian torsion, ovarian mass, dysmenorrhea, endometriosis, mittelschmerz (ovulatory pain)
- Urinary tract causes: Urinary tract infection, nephrolithiasis

- Gastrointestinal causes: Appendicitis, inflammatory bowel disease, gastroenteritis, mesenteric adenitis, constipation, Meckel diverticulum

■ Management
- Consider hospitalization when poor adherers, young adolescents, vomiting, ovarian abscess, and ectopic pregnancy or appendicitis not yet excluded
- Educate regarding STD prevention

Uncomplicated Cervicitis
- Ceftriaxone or ciprofloxacin (one dose) *plus* azithromycin (one dose) or doxycycline (BID for 7 days)

Pelvic Inflammatory Disease
- Inpatient therapy: IV cefoxitin or cefotetan *plus* doxycycline
  - Alternate: IV clindamycin plus gentamicin
  - At discharge: PO doxycycline to complete 14 days vs. clindamycin to complete 14 days (if tubo-ovarian abscess is present)
- Outpatient options: Ofloxacin (14 days) plus metronidazole (14 days)
  - Alternate: Ceftriaxone (one dose) plus doxycycline (14 days)

Complications
- Ectopic pregnancy, infertility, recurrent infection, tubo-ovarian abscess, chronic abdominal pain, and perihepatitis (Fitz-Hugh and Curtis syndrome)

Infectious Diseases in the Sexually Abused Child

■ Epidemiology/Risk Factors
- Low prevalence of STDs but certain situations warrant screening:
  - Children with symptomatic infection
  - Another STD diagnosed in the same child
  - Perpetrator or another sibling in the household found to have an STD
  - Assault has occurred within 24 to 48 hours and postexposure prophylaxis is considered
  - Clear evidence of injury or transfer of secretions from the perpetrator to the victim
  - All girls staged Tanner III or greater

■ Etiology
- *N. gonorrhoeae, C. trachomatis*, herpes simplex virus (HSV), HIV, syphilis, hepatitis B or C, *Trichomonas vaginalis*, human papilloma virus (HPV)

■ Laboratory Evaluation

- Vaginal rather than cervical cultures are appropriate for prepubertal children
- Recommended tests when screening sexually abused children for STDs:
  - Vaginal/rectal swab: Culture for *N. gonorrhoeae* and *C. trachomatis* (rapid detection techniques not validated in prepubertal children and should not be used in this setting); vaginal swab also for Gram stain and wet mount for *T. vaginalis*
  - Throat culture: *N. gonorrhoeae*
  - Serum: HIV antibodies (at time 0, 2, and 6 months), rapid plasmin reagin (syphilis), hepatitis B surface antigen, and hepatitis C antibodies (consider when significant tissue injury and high likelihood of transmission)
- If sexual contact has occurred within 72 hours, forensic evidence should be collected: 1) Rape kit, analyzed by the police laboratory; 2) clothing and bed linens collected in a paper bag; 3) Wood lamp to identify dried secretions (sample using moistened swab); 4) fingernail scrapings, when applicable; 5) saliva and blood from the victim

■ Management

- *N. gonorrhoeae*: Ceftriaxone (one dose)
- *C. trachomatis*: Azithromycin (one dose)
- Syphilis: Penicillin
- *T. vaginalis*: Metronidazole (3 days or one dose depending on age)
- Hepatitis B: Vaccinate if unimmunized
- HIV: Consider postexposure prophylaxis (see Chapter 21)

■ Medicolegal Interpretations

- In a child evaluated for suspected abuse, an STD diagnosis supports the investigation
- Occasionally, an STD is diagnosed but sexual abuse in not suspected. Potential problems for interpretation of test results include: 1) Many STDs vertically transmitted during birth; 2) some pathogens (HPV, *C. trachomatis*) may have long incubation periods; 3) HSV and *T. vaginalis* can be spread by autoinoculation or innocent transmission by close household contacts

13 Skin and Soft-Tissue Infections

Laura Gomez, MD and Stephen C. Eppes, MD

Impetigo

- Superficial skin infection characterized by honey-crusted exudates
- Bullous form characterized by single or clustered bullae

■ Epidemiology

- Mainly in infants and young children (usually ages 2 to 5 years)
- Can affect adolescents sporadically or in epidemics
- More than 70% of infections are nonbullous type

■ Risk Factors

- Breaks in skin associated with wounds, HSV, angular chelitis, insect bites, abrasions

■ Etiology

- *Staphylococcus aureus* predominates (children of all ages), especially in bullous form
- *Streptococcus pyogenes* (most common in preschoolers, unusual before age 2 years)

■ Pathogenesis

- Skin compromised by minor trauma permits invasion by pathogen
- In bullous form, localized toxin production (exfoliatoxin or epidermolytic toxins A and B) causes separation of upper layers of epidermis

■ History/Physical Examination

Nonbullous

- Pruritic, spreading skin lesions with honey-crusted exudates often on face and extremities
- Absent constitutional symptoms
- Tender, erythematous papules evolve into small vesicles. The vesicles crust centrally with a thick, yellow exudate

- Little to no pain or surrounding erythema
- 90% have regional adenopathy

Bullous
- Superficial, thin-walled, fluid-filled lesion of varying size surrounded by erythematous base
- May be single or clustered; may become purulent
- Main sites: Face, extremities, perineum, and periumbilical area

■ **Additional Studies**
- Culture of fluid swabbed from beneath crusted lesion or from intact blister

■ **Differential Diagnosis**
Nonbullous
- Nonbullous form: Contact dermatitis, viral (herpes simplex, varicella), fungal (dermatophytes), scabies (all may become secondarily impetiginized)

Bullous
- Neonates: Epidermolysis bullosa; bullous mastocytosis; herpetic infection; scalded skin syndrome; group B streptococcal infection; congenital syphilis
- Older children: Insect bites; burns; erythema multiforme; chronic bullous dermatitis of childhood; bullous pemphigoid

■ **Management**
- For localized nonbullous lesions: Topical 2% mupirocin (Bactroban) for 7 to 10 days
- Most bullous lesions resolve spontaneously and without scarring in approximately 2 weeks
- Systemic therapy for widespread lesions, periorbital lesions, evidence of deeper involvement (cellulitis, abscess formation), and severe cases; use oral (dicloxacillin, cephalexin, clindamycin, amoxicillin-clavulanic acid) or parenteral antistaphylococcal antibiotics (cefazolin, nafcillin) for 7 days (alternative agents: clindamycin or macrolides)

■ **Complications**
- Cellulitis in approximately 10%; recurrent disease secondary to nasal carriage of *S. aureus*
- Acute poststreptococcal glomerulonephritis with nephritogenic strains of *S. pyogenes*
  - Overall incidence 2% to 5%; occurs within 18 to 21 days from onset

Cellulitis

- Infection of skin with varying extension into subcutaneous tissues

■ Epidemiology/Risk Factors
- Preferentially involves the lower extremities
- Risk factors: Lymphedema, site of entry secondary to trauma/bites, obesity

■ Etiology
- Common: *S. pyogenes*, *S. aureus*
- Less common: group B *Streptococcus* (neonates), *Pseudomonas aeruginosa* (immunocompromised)
- Prevaccine era: *Haemophilus influenzae* type b caused facial cellulitis

■ Pathogenesis
- Three mechanisms of infection: 1) Local wound infection (most common); 2) local extension from an underlying infection (e.g., osteomyelitis); 3) hematogenous seeding from bacteremia

History
- Local erythema, warmth, and pain
- Constitutional symptoms common including fever, chills, malaise
- If secondary to wound infection: Preceding puncture wound, insect bite, laceration
- If hematogenous seeding: URI prodrome followed by fever with simultaneous appearance of local erythema

■ Physical Examination
- Tender, indurated, edematous area of subcutaneous tissue with overlying warmth and erythema
- Indistinct lateral margins secondary to process lying deep within subcutaneous tissue
- Regional lymphadenopathy and lymphangitic streaking

■ Additional Studies
- Culture of aspirate from site of inflammation
- Blood culture positive in less than 10%

■ Differential Diagnosis
- Deep venous thrombosis; ruptured baker's cyst; erythema nodosum; insect bites; septic arthritis; osteomyelitis

■ Management

- If constitutional symptoms (e.g., fever) absent: Oral therapy with penicillinase-resistant penicillin or first-generation cephalosporin. Consider clindamycin empirically in areas with high MRSA prevalence.
- Use parenteral therapy (oxacillin, nafcillin, or cefazolin) for fever, rapid progression lymphangitis, or lymphadenitis. Consider vancomycin in areas with high prevalence of methicillin-resistant *S. aureus*
- Add **antipseudomonal coverage** in severely immunocompromised and **for nail puncture** injuries

■ Complications

- Circumferential cellulitis: Swelling may cause neurovascular compromise requiring surgical decompression
- Cellulitis may represent deeper underlying infection (e.g., dental or sinus infection causing facial cellulitis, ischiorectal abscess with perianal cellulitis)

Folliculitis, Furuncles, and Carbuncles

- Many skin infections begin in the hair follicle resulting in local abscess formation
- Further classification is by depth of involvement of the hair follicle
  - Folliculitis: Small abscess with limited surrounding tissue reaction
  - Furuncle: Deeper nodule with more intense tissue reaction still involving a single follicle
  - Carbuncle: Multiseptate, loculated abscess; aggregate of infected hair follicles

■ Epidemiology/Risk Factors/Etiology

- Risk factors include wounds from injuries, bites, or surgery; hot tub use
- *S. aureus* predominates
- Hot tub folliculitis usually due to *P. aeruginosa*

■ Pathogenesis

- Heavy skin colonization with *S. aureus* favors development of folliculitis
- Portal of entry created by preceding site of skin trauma allows pathogen to invade

■ History/Physical Examination

- Preceding history of trauma, wound, irritation, hot tub use
- Pustules commonly found on extremities, buttocks, or scalp

- Folliculitis: Discrete, dome-shaped pustule with an erythematous base, systemic symptoms rare
- Furuncle: Tender, erythematous, fluctuant, firm mass; predilection for areas exposed to friction
- Carbuncle: Swollen, erythematous, deep, painful mass; fever more likely

■ Additional Studies

- Gram stain and culture of purulent material

■ Differential Diagnosis

- Folliculitis may resemble papulovesicular diseases (e.g., herpes zoster, insect bites)
- Insect or spider bites may mimic skin abscess with surrounding cellulitis

■ Management

- Local measures: **Warm compresses**
- For furuncles and carbuncles, surgical drainage may be necessary
- First line: Penicillinase-resistant antibiotic such as **dicloxacillin** or first-generation cephalosporin. Alternative: Clindamycin (especially in areas with high MRSA prevalence) or macrolides

■ Complications

- Frequent recurrences with some strains:
  - Prophylaxis against recurrences involves eradication of staphylococcal colonization
  - For example, combining topical bacitracin, nasal mupirocin, and oral antistaphylococcal penicillin (or clindamycin) plus rifampin, and chlorhexidine baths (for 3 to 7 days)
- Recurrent skin abscesses should prompt search for phagocyte defect (see Chapter 22)

Necrotizing Fasciitis

- Extensive cellulitis with severe involvement of subcutaneous tissue including fascia, muscle, or both resulting in tissue necrosis

■ Epidemiology/Risk Factors

- Type I: In patients with diabetes and peripheral vascular disease (mainly adults)
- Type II: All age groups including neonates

- Risk factors: Immunodeficiency, neutropenia, surgery, varicella, penetrating injury

■ Etiology

- Type I: Mixed aerobic (*S. aureus*, gram-negative enteric organisms, and *P. aeruginosa*) and anaerobic (*Peptostreptococcus*, *Bacteroides fragilis*) infections
- Type II: Group A *Streptococcus* (GAS) (most common)

■ Pathogenesis

- Following trauma, surgery, or other conditions, skin becomes portal of entry for GAS infection
- Hematogenous translocation of GAS from the throat to site of blunt trauma or muscle strain
- Pyrogenic exotoxins from GAS strains lead to cytokine production and tissue damage
- Infection spreads along fascial planes, eventually producing myonecrosis and gangrene

■ History/Physical Examination

- Antecedent wound or varicella; fever and prostration
- Erythema, edema, and tenderness with *pain disproportionate to physical findings*
- Overlying skin may develop blebs, bullae, and necrosis
- Fever, malaise, myalgias, anorexia may occur during first 24 hours
- Systemic complication due to shock and metabolic abnormalities may occur in advanced cases

■ Additional Studies

- CT or MRI of involved area allows assessment of extent of tissue involvement
- Blood cultures and cultures of skin/soft tissue lesions
- Direct surgical exploration allows definitive diagnosis and cultures

■ Differential Diagnosis

- Severe cellulitis; pyomyositis

■ Management

- Urgent surgical drainage and debridement, antibiotic therapy, hemodynamic supportive care
- Initial antibiotic therapy should provide coverage for aerobic and anaerobic organisms: Combination of clindamycin or penicillinase-resistant penicillin plus an aminoglycoside (e.g., gentamicin), or a

third-generation cephalosporin, or a β-lactam/β-lactamase inhibitor combination. If etiology is GAS, the combination of a β-lactam (penicillin or cephalosporin) and clindamycin is probably superior to the β-lactam alone (Eagle effect)
- In patients with streptococcal toxic shock, consider use of IVIG (neutralization of circulating streptococcal toxin; see Chapter 15 for toxic shock syndrome)

■ Complications
- Streptococcal toxic shock syndrome; loss of limb; death

Jane M. Gould, MD, FAAP

Septic Arthritis

- Microbial invasion of the synovial space

■ Epidemiology

- One third to one half of cases occur in children younger than 2 years
- 90% are monoarticular; large joints (knee > hip > ankle > elbow) most common overall
- Lyme affects knee in 90%; *Neisseria gonorrhoeae* affects distal joints (hands, wrists, knees)

■ Risk Factors

- Most children previously healthy
- Occasionally preexisting joint disease (e.g., rheumatoid arthritis) or impaired host defense (e.g., malignancies, primary immunodeficiency, steroids)

■ Etiology/Pathogenesis (Table 14-1)

- Three main mechanisms: 1) Hematogenous spread via synovial membrane (most common); 2) direct inoculation or puncture of joint space by contaminated object; 3) contiguous extension from an adjacent osteomyelitis in neonates and young infants

■ History

- Acute onset of fever, limp, refusal to walk, refusal to use limb
- Lyme arthritis may be preceded by erythema migrans rash; few systemic symptoms
- *N. gonorrhoeae* preceded by fever, chills, tenosynovitis, and polyarthralgias

■ Physical Examination

- Abduction and external rotation typical with hip involvement.
- Bacterial arthritis: Joint swelling, warmth, erythema, decreased mobility, exquisitely tender

■ TABLE 14-1 Etiology of Septic Arthritis

Age	Common	Less Common
Neonate	S. aureus Group B Streptococcus	N. gonorrhoeae Candida spp. Enteric GNR
Infant	S. aureus S. pyogenes K. kingae	S. pneumoniae H. influenzae[a] Salmonella spp.[b]
Older child/adolescent	S. aureus N. gonorrhoeae S. pyogenes	H. influenzae S. pneumoniae Salmonella spp.

[a] H. influenzae type b in unimmunized populations.
[b] Salmonella in patients with sickle cell disease.

- Lyme arthritis: Swelling and erythema out of proportion to tenderness
- N. gonorrhoeae: Hemorrhagic papules/pustules on extensor surfaces and over affected joints
- Multiple joints may be involved in gonococcal infection and in neonates

■ Additional Studies

- Blood cultures positive in 40% of cases.
- Joint aspiration of synovial fluid for culture positive in 50%
  - Yield increases when synovial fluid inoculated directly into blood culture bottle rather than onto agar plates (conventional method)
  - Also send Gram stain and cell count; usually more than 50,000 WBCs/mm^3 with more than 90% neutrophils
- Consider synovial fluid polymerase chain reaction for Lyme and N. gonorrhoeae when appropriate
- Urethral, rectal, or cervical cultures if N. gonorrhoeae suspected
- Radiographs: May see soft-tissue swelling, joint space widening, osteomyelitis
- Consider technetium bone scanning or MRI with contrast to diagnose contiguous osteomyelitis

■ Differential Diagnosis

- Reactive arthritis (Shigella, Salmonella, Yersinia, Campylobacter, Meningococcus, Chlamydia, Mycoplasma)
- Inflammatory conditions: Rheumatologic conditions (juvenile rheumatoid arthritis, collagen vascular diseases); acute rheumatic fever; inflammatory bowel disease; leukemia

- Hip pain: Toxic synovitis, psoas abscess, pelvic osteomyelitis, Legg-Calvé-Perthes disease, slipped capital femoral epiphysis, fracture

■ Management

- Empiric intravenous antibiotics (alter therapy based on organism isolated)
  - Neonate: Oxacillin/vancomycin + aminoglycoside/cefotaxime
  - Infant or child: Oxacillin/cefazolin/ceftriaxone (vancomycin if high methicillin-resistant *S. aureus* prevalence)
  - Adolescent: Consider ceftriaxone (for *N. gonorrhoeae*)
- Lyme: Initial amoxicillin or doxycycline (ceftriaxone for treatment failure)
- Duration of therapy varies by organism: Typical bacterial arthritis, 2 to 3 weeks; Lyme arthritis, 4 weeks; *N. gonorrhoeae*, 7 to 10 days. If associated osteomyelitis, duration as for osteomyelitis
- In older children *without* hip involvement or associated osteomyelitis, consider switching to oral therapy after clinical and laboratory improvement documented (consult infectious diseases specialist)
- Needle aspiration for all joints. Open surgical drainage and irrigation if 1) hip or shoulder involved; 2) persistent/recurrent symptoms; 3) penetrating joint injury; 4) neonatal patient

■ Complications

- Osteonecrosis; growth arrest; cartilage damage, stiff or unstable joint with poor mobility, chronic dislocation; sepsis

Osteomyelitis

- Infection of bone

■ Epidemiology

- Most (more than 50%) acute hematogenous osteomyelitis cases occur in the first 5 years of life
- Bones affected: Femur > tibia > humerus > hands/feet > pelvis > radius/ulna

■ Risk Factors

- Trauma: Open fractures, orthopedic surgery, decubitus ulcers, bites, IV drug abuse
- Vascular insufficiency: Sickle hemoglobinopathies, diabetes
- Extension of previous infection: Sinusitis, mastoiditis, dental abscess

---

■ BOX 14-1 Etiology of Osteomyelitis

Neonates
Group B Streptococcus
Staphylococcus aureus
Candida spp.
Enterobacteriaceae
Other streptococci

Infants
Staphylococcus aureus
Streptococcus pyogenes
Streptococcus pneumoniae
Kingella kingae
Haemophilus influenzae

Older Children
Staphylococcus aureus
Streptococcus pyogenes
Salmonella spp.

■ Etiology/Pathogenesis (Box 14-1)

- Three main mechanisms: 1) Hematogenous seeding (most common); 2) direct inoculation (e.g., puncture wound, following surgery); 3) contiguous spread
- Age-related differences in the anatomy of the bone and its blood supply influence clinical manifestations. In neonates and infants, osteomyelitis may spread to adjacent joint via trans-physeal vessels (these vessels recede by age 6 to 12 months)

■ History

- Symptoms, including fever, usually present for less than 2 weeks
- Most frequent manifestations include fever, pain at site of infection, and refusal to use limb
- Less common manifestations include anorexia, malaise, and vomiting

■ Physical Examination

- Limitation of use of involved extremity or area
- Localized swelling, warmth, erythema, and pain
- Special considerations
  - Pelvic osteomyelitis: Hip and/or abdominal pain, difficulty walking, rectal mass

- Vertebral osteomyelitis: Back pain, fever, usually older than 3 years, tenderness over spinal processes. Spinal radiographs are usually normal, but MRI reveals bony destruction
- *Pseudomonas* osteochondritis: Foot puncture wound followed by local findings after 3 to 4 days, fever is not prominent

■ Additional Studies

- ESR, CRP: Often elevated at presentation
- Blood cultures positive in 50% of cases
- Consider bone biopsy for histopathology and cultures
- X-rays: Can exclude fracture or bone tumor, but changes of osteomyelitis (periosteal new bone formation) usually not present until 2 weeks after symptoms begin
- Technetium bone scan: Especially useful for detecting multifocal disease
- MRI with contrast: Best imaging modality

■ Differential Diagnosis

- General: Child abuse/trauma; leukemia; skeletal neoplasia (Ewing sarcoma); bone infarction (sickle cell disease); cellulitis; thrombophlebitis
- Clavicle/vertebral/rib osteomyelitis: Chronic recurrent multifocal osteomyelitis

■ Management

- Antimicrobial therapy (Table 14-2)
- Indications for surgery: 1) Drainage of purulent material from subperiosteal space or adjacent tissues (sequestra); 2) removal of infected foreign material; 3) debridement of nonviable

■ TABLE 14-2 Therapy for Osteomyelitis[a]

Etiology	Recommended Agents	Duration
MSSA	Oxacillin/cefazolin/clindamycin	3–4 wk
MRSA	Vancomycin/linezolid	3–4 wk
Streptococci	Penicillin/ampicillin	3–4 wk
P. aeruginosa	Ticarcillin/piperacillin + aminoglycoside	7–10 d with debridement
Salmonella	Ampicillin (if sensitive)/cefotaxime/ceftriaxone/ TMP-SMZ	3–4 wk
K. kingae	Penicillin (if sensitive)/ cefotaxime/ceftriaxone/ TMP-SMZ	3–4 wk

[a] Specific therapy should be altered based on susceptibility testing.

tissue; 4) signs and symptoms fail to improve within 48 hours (clinical improvement is usually seen *before* radiographic improvement); 5) chronic osteomyelitis
- CRP usually peaks on second day of appropriate therapy and normalizes at 7 to 9 days. ESR typically peaks at 5 to 7 days and normalizes by 3 to 4 weeks after initiation of appropriate therapy

■ Complications
- Growth plate damage (most common in the neonate); septic arthritis
- Chronic osteomyelitis (usually develops when diagnosis and treatment have been delayed)

15 Bloodstream Infections

Arlene Dent, MD, PhD and John R. Schreiber, MD, MPH

Sepsis

- Systemic inflammatory response syndrome (SIRS): Describes the inflammatory response to an insult. May be infectious or noninfectious. Manifested by two or more of the following: hyper- or hypothermia, cardiac dysfunction, respiratory dysfunction, or perfusion abnormalities
- Sepsis: Infection plus systemic inflammatory response (e.g., fever, tachycardia, leukocytosis or leukopenia). "Severe" if associated with altered organ perfusion
- Septic shock: Severe sepsis plus hypotension despite adequate fluid resuscitation

■ Epidemiology/Risk Factors

- Bimodal distribution with peaks during neonatal period and at 2 years of age
- Young age, immune suppression (see Chapters 22 and 23), anatomic abnormality (e.g., urinary obstruction leading to urosepsis), invasive procedures (e.g., surgery), foreign body [e.g, central venous catheter (CVC)], malnutrition, traumatic/thermal wounds

■ Etiology (Box 15-1)

- Organisms vary by age. Hospitalized children are at risk for additional organisms

■ Pathogenesis

- Complex host responses determine the extent of inflammatory response
- Virulence factors (e.g., endotoxins or lipopolysaccharide for gram-negative rods) activate mechanisms involving complement, clotting, fibrinolytic, and kinin pathways
  - Proinflammatory cytokines released including TNF-α
  - Systemic activation of coagulation generates fibrin deposition in small blood vessels, causing microvascular thrombosis in critical organs and leading to organ failure
  - Consumption of clotting proteins leads to bleeding

■ BOX 15-1 Causes of Sepsis in Children

Neonates
Group B *Streptococcus*
Escherichia coli
Klebsiella spp.
Enterococcus spp.
Listeria monocytogenes
Viruses [a]

Infants/Older Children
Streptococcus pneumoniae
Neisseria meningitidis
Group A *Streptococcus*
Staphylococcus aureus
Haemophilus influenzae [b]

Nosocomial
Coagulase-negative staphylococci
Enterobacter spp.
Pseudomonas aeruginosa
Enteric gram-negative rods
Candida spp.
Staphylococcus aureus

[a] Especially herpes simplex virus and enteroviruses (e.g., coxsackie virus and echovirus).
[b] If unimmunized.

■ History/Physical Examination

- Fever, comorbidities, immunodeficiency, immunosuppressive medications, immunization status, travel, animal exposure, instrumentation
- Assess respiratory and hemodynamic stability and detect potential infection sources
- Common findings in sepsis: Hyper- or hypothermia, tachycardia, hypotension, tachypnea, pallor, evidence of altered organ perfusion, ecthyma, petechiae or purpura
- Additional findings: Cyanosis, oliguria, jaundice, congestive heart failure

■ Additional Studies

- Age and localizing signs direct initial workup (examination less reliable in infants)
    - Leukocytosis or leukopenia, thrombocytopenia
    - Respiratory alkalosis, lactic acidosis
    - Cultures of blood, urine, and CSF (if stable)
    - Elevated PT, PTT, fibrinogen split products, and D dimer

- Imaging studies to consider: CXR, head or abdominal CT, extremity MRI

■ **Differential Diagnosis**

- Metabolic/endocrine: Adrenal insufficiency, electrolyte disturbances, dehydration, diabetes insipidus, diabetes mellitus, inborn errors of metabolism
- Also, GI (volvulus, intussusception, hemorrhage); neurologic (intoxication, intracranial hemorrhage); Kawasaki; Stevens-Johnson; hemolytic-uremic syndrome

■ **Management**

- Specific antibiotic therapy depends on the source of the infection (e.g., meningitis, pneumonia; see specific topics for details of directed therapy)
- Empiric treatment:
  - **Neonate (early-onset sepsis):** Ampicillin + aminoglycoside or cefotaxime (consider adding acyclovir if herpes simplex virus suspected)
  - **Neonate (nosocomial sepsis):** Vancomycin + aminoglycoside + ceftazidime
  - **Child (previously healthy):** Cefotaxime or ceftriaxone, consider vancomycin (consider adding doxycycline in tick-endemic areas)
  - **Child (nosocomial sepsis):** Vancomycin + gram-negative coverage taking into account hospital resistance patterns (consider aminoglycosides, third-generation cephalosporins, extended-spectrum penicillins, or carbapenems)
  - Alter therapy based on patient comorbidities, local resistance patterns, culture results and susceptibility testing (see Chapter 3 for spectrum of antimicrobial agents)
- Recombinant activated protein C (rhAPC; Xigris):
  - Up to 80% of children and adults with severe sepsis develop acquired protein C deficiency (associated with shock and death) during sepsis-induced coagulopathy.
  - Proposed mechanism of action: 1) Antithrombotic (inactivates factors Va and VIIIa); 2) profibrinolytic (inactivates plasminogen activator-1); 3) anti-inflammatory (inhibits thrombin and cytokine formation)
  - In adults, 19.4% reduction in relative risk of mortality. One additional life was saved for every 16 patients treated. Patients at high risk of bleeding excluded from study
  - Sparse data in children but trials ongoing

■ **Complications**

- Multiple organ dysfunction; death rate ranges from 5% to 50%

Central Venous Catheter-Related Infections

- CVC devices range from peripherally inserted central catheters (PICCs) to tunneled CVCs to implanted multilumen plastic catheters
- Infections range from localized infections (exit site, tunnel tract, and suppurative phlebitis) to systemic infections (bacteremia and fungemia)

■ Epidemiology

- Incidence of exit site infection is 0.2 to 2.8 per 1000 catheter-days
- Incidence of CVC sepsis is 1.7 to 2.4 per 1000 catheter-days
- Incidence of implantable device sepsis is 0.3 to 1.8 per 1000 catheter-days

■ Risk Factors

- Depend on the device/product inserted, insertion site, and duration of CVC insertion
- Higher rates in 1) premature infants compared to older children; 2) intensive care units compared to general wards; 3) those receiving certain infusates (e.g., parenteral nutrition, contaminated fluids)

■ Etiology/Pathogenesis (Box 15-2)

- Interpretation of contaminant vs. pathogen affected by age and comorbidities.
- Routes of infection: 1) Inoculation at time of CVC placement; 2) inoculation during CVC manipulation (breach in aseptic

---

■ BOX 15-2 Causes of CVC-Related Infections[a]

Common Organisms
Coagulase-negative staphylococci
Staphylococcus aureus
Aerobic gram-negative bacilli
Candida albicans

Less Common Organisms
Corynebacterium species
Bukholderia cepacia
Stenotrophomonas maltophilia
Mycobacterium species

[a] In the neonate, the most common organisms causing infection are coagulase-negative staphylococci > *Candida* spp. > enterococci > gram-negative bacilli.

technique allows catheter colonization followed by infection); 3) hematogenous seeding (follows transient bacteremia); 4) extension of local infection (less common)

■ History/Physical Examination
- Fever without clear source of infection in presence of a CVC
- Local infection (confined to exit site): Erythema, tenderness, or purulent discharge
- Signs of systemic illness

■ Additional Studies
- Local infection: Gram stain and culture of any purulent discharge from exit site
- Systemic infection: Blood cultures from the catheter and a peripheral vein
  - CVC-related infection if 1) quantitative blood culture with 5:1 ratio or higher (CVC vs. peripheral) of colony count or 100 cfu/mL or higher from CVC culture; 2) differential time to positivity (e.g., positive result of culture from CVC appears 2 hours or more before positive result from peripheral culture; or 3) same organism from CVC and peripheral blood sample and 15 cfu or more of that organism from CVC tip

■ Differential Diagnosis
- Sepsis, cellulitis, phlebitis, drug-related fever, viral infection

■ Management (Table 15-1)
- Decision to remove CVC depends on 1) severity of the patient's condition; 2) evidence of catheter-related infection; 3) type of organism infecting the device
  - *Must* remove catheter if 1) candidemia; 2) *S. aureus* infection; 3) persistently positive blood cultures despite antimicrobial therapy; 4) tunnel infection
- Start antimicrobial therapy after obtaining blood cultures
  - Empiric: Combination therapy with oxacillin or vancomycin plus an aminoglycoside or third-generation cephalosporin. Alternate options include monotherapy with imipenem, meropenem, or cefepime (methicillin-resistant *Staphylococcus aureus* is not covered with this regimen)
- CVC-related candidemia: CVC removal plus antifungal therapy
  - Empiric antifungal therapy: Amphotericin B or liposomal derivative (see Chapter 4)

■ TABLE 15-1 Approach to Management of Uncomplicated Central Venous Catheter–Related Infection

Organism	Duration (days)[a]	Comments
CoNS	10–14	May retain CVC unless clinical deterioration or persisting or relapsing bacteremia. If catheter removed, may shorter duration of treatment to 5–7 days
S. aureus	14	Remove CVC; If echocardiogram reveals vegetations, treat for 4–6 weeks
Enterococcus	10–14	Usually treated with combination of vancomycin, ampicillin, or penicillin plus an aminoglycoside
GNR	10–14	Consider CVC removal for persistent positive cultures or clinical deterioration
Candida spp.	14	Remove CVC. Consider evaluation for dissemination
Mycobacteria	Unclear	Remove catheter. If peripheral blood cultures positive, may require more than 6 weeks of treatment

[a] Duration of therapy varies depending on presence of complications and specific underlying disease conditions. Optimal duration of therapy has not been established in children. Recommendations are extrapolated from adult data.

- Fluconazole may be used if the organism is susceptible.
- Evaluation includes routine ophthalmologic exam. For persistently positive cultures, consider echocardiogram, abdominal ultrasound or CT, and head CT

■ Complications

- Endocarditis, septic thrombosis, tunnel infections, and metastatic seeding
- If complications occur, antimicrobial duration may have to be extended or changed

Toxic Shock Syndrome

- Toxic shock syndrome (TSS): An acute febrile illness primarily caused by bacterial exotoxins. Patients with features of TSS but not meeting criteria (see "Physical Examination") can have a toxin-mediated process that is generally less severe

■ Epidemiology

- 10–20 cases per 100,000 population

■ Risk Factors/Etiology

- Menstruation and tampon use (*Staphylococcus aureus*); varicella (*S. pyogenes*)

■ Pathogenesis

- *S. aureus* strains can produce exotoxin (TSS toxin-1) and enterotoxins
- *S. pyogenes* strains can produce at least one of five pyrogenic exotoxins

■ History/Physical Examination

- *Major criteria (all required):* 1) Fever (greater than 38.9°C); 2) diffuse macular erythrodermatous rash that desquamates 1 to 2 weeks after disease onset. Can localize to the trunk, extremities, or perineum; 3) hypotension
- *Minor criteria (any three):* Vomiting, diarrhea, liver dysfunction, renal dysfunction, respiratory dysfunction (including ARDS), CNS changes, mucous membrane inflammation (hyperemia of the pharynx, tongue, and conjunctiva), and muscle abnormalities (including myocarditis)
- *S. aureus* more commonly associated with profuse diarrhea and foreign body at site of infection. *S. pyogenes* more commonly associated with localized soft-tissue infection (e.g., cellulitis, necrotizing fasciitis)

■ Additional Studies

- CBC with differential (leukocytosis or leukopenia, anemia, and thrombocytopenia)
- Blood culture positive for *S. aureus* in less than 5% of infected patients
- Cultures of foreign bodies and abscesses
- Throat rapid antigen test and culture for *S. pyogenes*
- *S. aureus* colonization screens can be performed but are not necessary
- Increased ASO or antiDNAase B 4 to 6 weeks after infection may confirm diagnosis
- Other findings: Hyponatremia, hypokalemia, hypocalcemia, hyperbilirubinemia (75%), elevated creatinine kinase (60%; rhabdomyolysis)
- Urinanalysis: Sterile pyuria, myoglobinuria, red blood cell casts
- Imaging to detect focal infection: CXR, abdominal CT, bone scan, or extremity MRI

■ Differential Diagnosis

- Infectious: Meningococcemia, Rocky Mountain spotted fever, ehrlichiosis, measles, staphylococcal scalded skin syndrome, scarlet fever, leptospirosis
- Noninfectious: Kawasaki, systemic lupus erythematosus, Stevens-Johnson syndrome

■ Management

- Supportive care, consider intensive care unit setting
  - Search for localized infection, remove foreign bodies (e.g., tampons), send cultures.
- Empiric therapy: β-Lactam antibiotic (oxacillin, nafcillin or cefazolin). Use vancomycin in place of β-lactam if patient unstable or deteriorating
  - Add clindamycin for severe disease because it may suppress toxin synthesis.
  - Adjust antimicrobial therapy based on culture results
- Duration of antimicrobial therapy: 10 to 14 days. Oral therapy once patient is stable
- Consider IVIG or corticosteroids for severe illness.

■ Complications

- Multiorgan failure; death (less than 3% with *S. aureus* but 30% to 70% with *S. pyogenes*)

16 Trauma-Related Infections

Reza J. Daugherty, MD and Dennis R. Durbin, MD, MSCE

Infections Following Trauma

■ Epidemiology

- Infection follows 1% to 2% of lacerations and 20% to 40% of major trauma

■ Risk Factors

- Simple laceration infection: Soil contamination; more than 3 cm length; foreign body
- Hospitalized major trauma infection: Invasive procedures; indwelling catheters; prolonged hospitalization; spinal cord injury; mechanical ventilation

■ Etiology

- For simple lacerations: *Staphylococcus aureus* and Group A *Streptococcus*
- In major trauma victims, most (75%) infections are nosocomial (Table 16-1)

■ Pathogenesis

- Breaks in skin and mucosal barriers allow pathogens to gain entry
- Devitalized tissue harbors pathogens not accessible to the immune system
- Major trauma impairs humoral and cellular immunity

■ TABLE 16-1 Common Infections and Organisms in Hospitalized Major Trauma Patients

Site of Infection	Organisms
Respiratory tract	S. aureus, H. influenzae, P. aeruginosa
Urinary system	E. coli, Enterococcus spp., P. aeruginosa
Bloodstream	Coagulase-negative staphylococci, S. aureus
Surgical wound	S. aureus, P. aeruginosa
Soft tissue	S. aureus
Abdomen	S. aureus, E. coli

■ Management

Lacerations

- Minor lacerations: Topical antimicrobial agents: Bacitracin or "triple antibiotic"; PO/IV antibiotic prophylaxis not usually required
- Tetanus immunization: Administer if patient received less than three doses of toxoid or unknown immunization status
  - Tetanus immunization *not* required for 1) clean minor wounds and three previous doses of toxoid less than 10 years before; 2) all other wounds and three previous doses of toxoid less than 5 years ago
- Tetanus immune globulin (TIG): Administer if contaminated wound and immunization status uncertain or less than three previous doses of toxoid
  - TIG *not* required for 1) clean minor wounds regardless of immunization status; 2) all other wounds and three previous doses of toxoid

Major Trauma

- Associated lacerations as above; antibiotic prophylaxis (Table 16-2).

■ Complications

- Mortality (10% to 20% in hospitalized major trauma patients); prolonged hospitalization

■ TABLE 16-2 Antibiotic Prophylaxis by Trauma Type

Type of Trauma	Antibiotic Prophylaxis
Oral trauma	Generally *not* required
Basilar skull fracture	Generally *not* required
Facial fracture	Cefazolin
Penetrating brain injury	Ceftriaxone
Penetrating thoracic injury	Cefazolin **or** oxacillin
Penetrating abdominal injury	Ampicillin/sulbactam
Multisystem trauma	Cefoxitin **or** ampicillin/sulbactam
Open extremity fractures	
Type I and II	Cefazolin **or** oxacillin
Type III	Cefazolin **or** oxacillin **and** gentamicin
Fecal contamination	
FHAL contamination (e.g., farm-related injury)	Add high-dose penicillin to above regimens

Infections Following Bites

■ **Epidemiology**

- Bites most commonly occur by dogs (80% to 90%), cats (5% to 15%), and humans (5%)
- Frequency of infection: Dog bite (2% to 20%); human bite (10% to 50%); cat bite (30% to 50%)
- High risk of rabies from bats (most common), raccoons, skunks, foxes, and coyotes
- Low risk of rabies from small rodents and lagomorphs

■ **Risk Factors**

- Risk factors for infection from bite wounds: 1) Location on hand/foot; 2) treatment delay more than 12 hours; 3) closed-fist punch to human mouth; 4) puncture wounds; 5) crush injury; 6) immunosuppression; 7) cat bites
- Risk factors for rabies: 1) Unprovoked attack, 2) high-risk animal (see "Epidemiology"), 3) unimmunized dog or cat, 4) unusual animal behavior

■ **Etiology**

- Frequently polymicrobial (three to five species) and usually contain anaerobes
  - Aerobes: *S. aureus, Streptococcus* spp., *Corynebacterium* spp.; anaerobes: *Bacteroides fragilis, Prevotella* spp., *Peptostreptococcus, Fusobacterium* spp.
  - From dogs/cats, also *Pasteurella* and *Capnocytophaga* species. From humans, also *Eikenella corrodens*
- Rabies (10 to 90 day incubation period)

■ **History/Physical Examination**

- Document type of animal, health of animal, provoked or unprovoked attack
- Determine if history of immunosuppression, asplenia, and tetanus immunization
- Determine wound type (laceration, avulsion, puncture), involvement of underlying structures (e.g., joint, cranial contents), neurovascular function
- Signs/symptoms: Fever, local erythema/edema, lymphangitic streaking, regional adenopathy, and purulent drainage. Sepsis possible
- Specific organisms: Pain and swelling within 12 to 24 hours (*Pasteurella*); rapid onset of sepsis and disseminated intravascular coagulation (*Capnocytophaga canimorsus*); indolent infection

after clenched fist injury (*E. corrodens*); anxiety, dysphagia, and seizures (rabies)

■ Management

General

- If infection present, obtain anaerobic and aerobic cultures. If fever, culture blood
- High-pressure irrigation, except for puncture wounds; debride devitalized tissue
- Tetanus immunization as with other minor wounds. Role of HIV prophylaxis unclear

Antibiotics

- Indications for antibiotic prophylaxis: 1) Puncture wounds, 2) bites on face or hand, 3) cat bite, 4) devitalized tissue, 5) crush injury, 6) immunocompromised patient
- Prophylactic antibiotic choice: Amoxicillin-clavulanate for 5 days
  - Alternate: TMP-SMX *and* clindamycin; cefotaxime; or ceftriaxone

Rabies

- Dogs and cats (if dog/cat unable to be observed, consult local public health official)
  - If healthy, observe for 10 days: Immunize patient if animal develops rabies
  - If signs/symptoms of rabies: Immunize patient *plus* rabies immune globulin (RIG)
- Other animals: Consider sacrifice to test brain tissue for rabies
  - For high-risk animals, rabies immunization and RIG unless animal tests negative
  - For low-risk animals, no specific prophylaxis
- Use either rabies human diploid cell vaccine (HDCV) or primary chick embryo cell vaccine. Previously unimmunized patients require doses on days 0, 3, 7, 14, and 28, whereas those with prior immunization only require doses on days 0 and 3

■ Complications

- Cellulitis, tenosynovitis, septic arthritis/osteomyelitis, sepsis, meningitis, endocarditis

Infections Following Burns

Epidemiology

- Burn victims: One third to one half are pediatric patients
- Incidence density of approximately 50 infections per 1000 hospital days

■ **Risk Factors**

- Full-thickness burns; more than 25% body surface area (BSA) affected; smoke inhalation; prolonged hospitalization; indwelling catheters; extremes of age; hyperglycemia

■ **Etiology**

- Infections frequently polymicrobial
- Wound infection: *S. aureus, Pseudomonas aeruginosa,* group A *Streptococcus, Enterobacter* spp., *Klebsiella* spp., *Enterococcus* spp., *Acinetobacter* spp.
- Bloodstream infection: Coagulase-negative staphylococci, *S. aureus, P. aeruginosa,* group *A Streptococcus, Klebsiella* spp.
- Pneumonia: *Streptococcus pneumoniae, S. aureus* (usually in ventilated patients)
- Urinary tract infections: *P. aeruginosa, Escherichia coli* (usually with urinary catheters)

■ **Pathogenesis**

- Significant burn injury leads to loss of normally protective skin barrier, decreased production of interferon-γ, immunoglobulins, and phagocytes, poor opsonic and bactericidal activity, and increased anergy to antigens
- Colonization of burn wounds occurs by spread of normal skin flora, translocation of gut flora, and nosocomial acquisition

■ **History/Physical Examination**

- Local: Edema, erythema, discoloration, or necrosis around wound edge; unexpectedly rapid eschar separation; hemorrhage under subeschar tissue; purulent exudates
- Systemic: Fever; hypothermia; hypotension; altered mentation

■ **Additional Studies**

- Histology (biopsy specimen): Bacteria, thrombosis or necrosis, intense inflammation
- Microbiology (biopsy specimen): Quantitative Gram stain and culture (more than 10^5 colonies per gram of tissue suggests infection)
- Blood cultures positive in 50% with systemic signs of infection

■ **Management**

- Prevention
  - Clean wound and debride necrotic tissue immediately
  - Dressings: Sterile gauze with elastic wrap, cadaveric allograft, porcine xenograft, or synthetic materials (e.g., Transcyte, Biobrane, etc.).

- - Indications for dressings: First degree, dressing not required; second degree, twice-daily dressing changes; third degree, autografting
- Tetanus passive immunization for inadequately immunized or unknown status
- Antibiotics
  - Topical antimicrobial agents indicated: Silver sulfadiazine (most common), mafenide acetate, polymyxin B, neomycin, or mupirocin
  - Systemic antibiotic prophylaxis *not* required unless grafting or excision performed
  - Empiric antibiotics for *suspected infection*: Gentamicin plus either ceftazidime, ticarcillin-clavulanate, imipenem, or ciprofloxacin plus an aminoglycoside
- Parenteral glutamine may decrease gram-negative sepsis; IVIG with unproven but potential benefit; interferon-γ not shown to reduce infection

■ Complications
- Increased hospitalization length, morbidity, and mortality; worse cosmetic outcome

17 Congenital/Perinatal Infections

Matthew J. Bizzarro, MD and Patrick G. Gallagher, MD

Approach to Congenital Infections

■ Etiology

- The major congenital infections are encompassed in the acronym TORCHES
  - Toxoplasmosis, Others, Rubella, Cytomegalovirus, Herpes simplex virus, Enterovirus, Syphilis
  - "Others": *Listeria monocytogenes*, varicella, human immunodeficiency virus (HIV), parvovirus, enteroviruses

■ Pathogenesis

- Fetal infection occurs by 1) transplacental passage (hematogenous spread; most common), 2) invasion through intact, damaged, or ruptured amniotic membranes, 3) exposure to infected maternal genital tract

■ Additional Studies

- Chorionic villus, amniotic fluid, and cord blood sampling allow in utero diagnosis
- Blood: IgM (toxoplasma, rubella), RPR (syphilis), hepatitis B surface antigen
- CSF: DNA PCR (enterovirus, HSV), Venereal Disease Research Laboratory (VDRL; syphilis)
- Skin lesions: DFA (HSV, varicella), dark field (syphilis)
- Viral culture: Conjunctiva (HSV), mouth (HSV, enterovirus), rectum (HSV, enterovirus), urine (CMV)
- Radiography of long bones (rubella, syphilis) or head CT (CMV, toxoplasmosis)
- Ophthalmologic exam (toxoplasmosis, rubella, CMV, HSV, syphilis, varicella)
- Hearing screen (rubella, CMV, toxoplasmosis)
- Other studies: Liver function tests, CBC

Congenital Toxoplasmosis

■ Epidemiology

- 39% of pregnant women in United States have *Toxoplasma* IgG antibodies
- In neonates, the rate of congenital infection is 1 to 3 per 1000 live births

■ Risk Factors

- Maternal ingestion of raw or undercooked meat containing *Toxoplasma* cysts
- Maternal exposure to oocysts in cat feces (litter boxes, sandboxes, gardens)

■ Etiology

- Caused by an intracellular, protozoan parasite, *Toxoplasma gondii*

■ Pathogenesis

- Infected cat then sheds oocysts in stool. Maternal infection occurs by ingestion of stool oocysts or undercooked meat containing cysts
- Congenital infection occurs via transplacental transmission. Risk of transmission during a primary infection is 40%

■ History/Physical Examination (also see "Risk Factors")

- Premature delivery (25% to 50% of affected infants) or symmetric intrauterine growth retardation (IUGR)
- In 70% to 90% of infants disease is asymptomatic at birth, but if symptomatic: Fever, seizures, jaundice, hydrocephalus, lymphadenopathy, hepatosplenomegaly, petechial/maculopapular rash

■ Additional Studies

- Neuroimaging: Hydro-/microcephaly; diffuse, intraparenchymal calcifications
- Ophthalmologic exam: Chorioretinitis
- Hearing screen: Sensorineural hearing loss
- CSF: Elevated protein and/or pleocytosis
- Blood: Indirect hyperbilirubinemia, pancytopenia

■ Diagnosis

- Neonatal IgM- or IgA-specific serum antibodies or persistently positive IgG titers

- Isolation of parasite from placenta, cord blood, neonatal blood, CSF, and/or urine
- PCR for DNA in CSF or peripheral blood leukocytes

■ Management

- Pyrimethamine, sulfadiazine, and folinic acid for 1 year
- Prenatal treatment (spiramycin) does not affect transmission rates but decreases incidence and severity of neonatal sequelae

■ Complications

- Progressive visual loss in two thirds of infected infants with chorioretinitis
- Severe disease: 10% mortality; survivors often have seizures or cerebral palsy
- Neonates with symptomatic disease may present later with impaired vision or learning

Congenital Syphilis

■ Epidemiology

- U.S. epidemic during 1990s. Improved prenatal care contributed to declining rates
- Incidence by race: African American > Hispanic > white

■ Risk Factors

- STD risk factors including HIV infection and multiple anonymous sexual partners

■ Etiology

- Caused by *Treponema pallidum*, a fastidious and motile spirochete

■ Pathogenesis

- Transmitted hematogenously (most cases) or via direct contact with infected mucocutaneous lesions during delivery
- Rate of transmission is 60% to 90% during untreated primary or secondary maternal syphilis but decreases to 10% to 30% in latent syphilis

■ History/Physical Examination

- Untreated or inadequately treated maternal infection: Pregnancy complicated by spontaneous abortion, hydrops fetalis, enlarged placenta, and/or premature delivery
- Subdivided into early (symptoms within the first 2 years of life) and late (more than 2 years) disease. Early manifestations

are due to active infection and inflammation whereas late manifestations are a consequence of scars induced by initial lesions of early congenital syphilis. Most with early syphilis diagnosed at 3 to 8 weeks of life

- *Early* disease: Low birth weight, failure to thrive, hydrocephalus, mucocutaneous bullous lesions, bloody rhinitis ("**snuffles**"), respiratory distress, generalized lymphadenopathy, hepatosplenomegaly, edema, osteochondritis, fever, and jaundice
- *Late* disease: Frontal bossing, saddle nose, scaphoid scapulas, **saber shins** (anterior bowing), mulberry molars (multicuspid first molars), **Hutchinson teeth** (peg-shaped upper incisors), rhagades (linear scars from corners of mouth), seizures

■ Additional Studies

- Radiography: "Celery stick" pattern of distal long bones (periosteal reaction/osteitis); diffuse pulmonary infiltrates (pneumonia alba)
- Neuroimaging: Optic atrophy on MRI
- Hearing screen: Sensorineural hearing loss
- CSF: Elevated protein, pleocytosis, positive VDRL results
- Blood: Elevated bilirubin and transaminases, hemolysis, leukocytosis, low platelets

■ Diagnosis

- Nontreponemal: VDRL, rapid plasma reagin (RPR), automated reagin test in serum and VDRL in CSF; high false positives with concomitant infections like VZV, EBV, and TB
- Treponemal: Fluorescent treponemal antibody absorption test (FTA-ABS) and microhemagglutination for *Treponema pallidum* (MHA-TP): detect antibodies to membrane proteins of *T. pallidum*; used to confirm a positive VDRL or RPR
- Identification of spirochetes on dark-field microscopy or by DFA of exudates from lesions or infected tissue (e.g., placenta or umbilical cord)

■ Management

- All newborn infants require nontreponemal antibody test prior to discharge
- Infants require further evaluation if mother has one or more of the following: 1) Unmanaged or undocumented management of syphilis; 2) syphilis during pregnancy managed with non-penicillin (non-PCN) antibiotics; 3) appropriately managed syphilis without a decrease in antibody titers; 4) syphilis managed less than 30 days prior to delivery; or 5) syphilis managed prior to pregnancy without sufficient follow-up titers

- Neonatal evaluation should then include *quantitative* nontreponemal and treponemal serologic tests
- Treat infant with aqueous crystalline or procaine PCN G for 10 days if 1) physical, laboratory, or radiographic evidence of infection; 2) positive dark-field test; 3) reactive CSF VDRL; or 4) infant's serum titers are fourfold greater than mother's
- Serologic testing in *treated* neonates should be performed at 2, 4, 6, and 12 months with titers undetectable by 6 months of age. If titers fail to decline or are present at 1 year, treat with aqueous crystalline PCN G for 10 to 14 days.

■ Complications

- Intrauterine death in 25% of pregnancies in mothers with early syphilis who have not received treatment. If live born, 25% to 30% die in the newborn period
- Survivors: Sensorineural deafness, blindness, retardation, and facial deformities

Congenital Rubella

■ Epidemiology

- In the United States, 20,000 cases in 1964/1965. Now fewer than 10 per year due to rubella vaccination

■ Risk Factors

- Unvaccinated populations and primary maternal infection in the first trimester

■ Etiology

- RNA virus of the Togaviridae family. Humans are only source of the virus

■ Pathogenesis

- Risk of vertical transmission from a mother with primary infection: first trimester: 80%; second trimester, 10% to 20%; third trimester, 25% to 50%
- Congenital malformations in 90% if infection occurs at less than 11 weeks gestation but only in 10% if 13th through 14th week gestation

■ History/Physical Examination

- Mother with susceptible rubella status on prenatal screening; spontaneous abortion
- 50% to 70% of infected neonates asymptomatic at birth

- Findings in symptomatic infants: Symmetric IUGR, seizures, large anterior fontanel, hydro- or microcephaly, hepatosplenomegaly, lymphadenopathy, patent ductus or pulmonary artery or valve stenosis, jaundice, purpuric **"blueberry muffin"** skin rash.

■ Additional Studies

- Radiography: Osteitis on long-bone films ("celery stalking")
- Neuroimaging: Intracranial calcifications on CT/MRI
- Ophthalmologic exam: **Cataract,** glaucoma, retinopathy
- Hearing screen: Sensorineural **hearing loss**
- Blood: Hyperbilirubinemia, transaminitis, hemolysis, **thrombocytopenia**

■ Diagnosis

- Virus-specific IgM from fetal or neonatal blood
- Culture of virus from the amniotic fluid, urine, blood, CSF, and/or nasopharynx
- Stable or increasing rubella-specific IgG over the first year of life

■ Management

- No antiviral treatment available; infected neonates require contact isolation

■ Complications

- Death (10% to 15%), autism, behavioral disorders, mental retardation, motor deficits, deafness (more than 80% of cases), glaucoma, diabetes mellitus, and thyroid abnormalities

Congenital Cytomegalovirus

■ Epidemiology

- Most common congenital viral infection
- Primary maternal infection occurs in 0.7% to 4.1% of pregnancies
- Transplacental transmission to fetus in 40% of primary maternal infections
- Most transplacentally infected infants have asymptomatic infection and develop normally; 10% to 15% of infected infants have symptomatic infection, and most (90%) of these have serious sequelae

■ Risk Factors

- Low socioeconomic group, young maternal age, and exposure to young children

■ Etiology

- The largest virus of the Herpesvirus family, double-stranded DNA

■ Pathogenesis

- Acquired via transplacental, intrapartum (passage through infected maternal genital tract), and postpartum (infected breast milk or blood transfusion) transmission
- First-trimester maternal primary infection most likely to result in fetal sequelae
- Predilection of virus for CNS, reticuloendothelial system, and liver

■ History/Physical Examination

- Pregnancy complicated by premature delivery or symmetric IUGR
- If symptomatic, findings include petechiae or purpura (75%), jaundice (65%), hepatosplenomegaly (60%), microcephaly (50%), and hypotonia (25%)

■ Additional Studies

- Radiography: Interstitial pneumonitis on CXR
- Neuroimaging: Microcephaly with ventriculomegaly, **periventricular calcifications**
- Ophthalmologic exam: Chorioretinitis
- Hearing screen: **Sensorineural hearing loss**
- Blood: Direct hyperbilirubinemia, elevated ALT, hemolysis, thrombocytopenia

■ Diagnosis

- Maternal infection: CMV-IgM and IgG (paired) antibody testing
- CMV detection in amniotic fluid or infant urine, peripheral blood leukocytes, or saliva within 3 weeks of birth: 1) Tissue culture (2 weeks), 2) rapid, centrifugation-enhanced culture (shell vial) using monoclonal antibody to early antigens (24 hours), or 3) DNA PCR (24–48 hours)
- Neonatal CMV IgG reflects past maternal infection; IgM not as sensitive as culture.

■ Management

- Treatment generally supportive, but in one study ganciclovir treatment of those with symptomatic congenital CMV and CNS disease reduced progression of hearing loss

- Hearing tests recommended every 3 months for the first year of life and then varies based on the presence or absence of findings

■ Complications

- 15% to 30% of newborns with symptomatic infection die in the newborn period
- 50% to 90% of surviving neonates with symptomatic infection have CNS impairment, including mental retardation, cerebral palsy, and visual abnormalities
- Progressive hearing loss in 50% of patients with symptomatic infection and 5% of patients with asymptomatic infection

Neonatal Herpes Simplex Virus Infection

- Types of maternal HSV infection
  - Primary: First infection with HSV in individual without previous HSV infection
  - Recurrent: Infection in an individual with previous HSV infection of same type/location
  - Nonprimary, first episode: First infection with HSV-1 in an individual with previous HSV-2 infection or vice versa

■ Epidemiology

- Neonatal infection in 1 in 3000 to 20,000 live births: 5% congenital, 95% intrapartum
- Site of intrapartum infection: Skin, eye, mucous membrane (34%); CNS (34%); disseminated (32%) (see below for details)

■ Risk Factors

- Symptomatic primary infection with vaginal delivery; Prolonged membrane rupture (more than 4 hours); prematurity; instrumentation (e.g., scalp electrodes)

■ Etiology

- HSV-1 causes 30% of neonatal infections and HSV-2 causes 70%

■ Pathogenesis

- Congenital infection: Acquisition during pregnancy from hematogenous spread
- Intrapartum transmission: Prenatally via vertical transmission through intact or ruptured membranes or perinatally via contact with infected maternal GU tract

- Neonatal infection occurs after vaginal delivery in 35% to 50% exposed to primary maternal infection vs. 3% to 5% exposed to recurrent maternal infection
- Primary infection has higher viral load, longer viral shedding period, and decreased amount of protective antibodies to be passed to the neonate
- Postpartum transmission: Postnatally via contact with active lesions (rare)

■ History

- Known maternal infection or vesicular lesions at delivery
- 60% to 80% of infected infants born to asymptomatic mothers

■ Physical Examination

- Onset varies from birth to 3 weeks of life **(typically at 11 to 17 days)** but 9% present within 24 hours of birth. Disseminated cases present earlier than CNS cases
- Congenital disease: Vesicles, scars, depigmented lesions at birth, microcephaly, seizures, abnormal neurologic examination, hepatosplenomegaly
- Skin/eye/mucous membranes: Vesicles at sites of trauma (scalp), oropharyngeal lesions, conjunctivitis, keratitis, chorioretinitis, cataracts
- CNS disease with or without vesicles: Lethargy, irritability seizures, vesicles (60%)
- Disseminated disease (involves multiple organs including CNS or skin): Respiratory distress, seizures, petechiae, disseminated intravascular coagulation, and vesicles

■ Additional Studies

- Radiography: Pneumonia begins centrally and involves entire lung in 1 to 3 days
- CSF: Elevated protein, low glucose, **lymphocytic pleocytosis** (50 to 100 WBC/mm^3)
- Blood: Elevated transaminases, coagulopathy, thrombocytopenia

■ Diagnosis

- Culture of vesicles, urine, stool/rectum, conjunctiva, mouth/nasopharynx, blood, CSF
  - Cultures of conjunctiva, mouth, and rectum positive in more than 90% with neonatal HSV
- DFA or EIA of vesicles for HSV antigen (rapid and 80% to 90% sensitivity)
- Tzank smear (low sensitivity; rarely used)
- CSF HSV PCR (best study to detect CNS involvement)

■ **Management**

- Acyclovir:
  - Skin/eye/mucous membrane disease: 60 mg/kg/d IV divided into three doses for 14 days
  - CNS/disseminated disease: 60 mg/kg/d IV divided into three doses for 21 days
  - Consider suppressive acyclovir for those with recurrent skin lesions
- Symptomatic neonate: Cultures and CSF PCR immediately, IV acyclovir
- Vaginal birth (primary infection): Cultures and CSF PCR at 24 to 48 hours, acyclovir
- Vaginal birth (recurrent infection): Surface cultures at 24 to 48 hours, IV acyclovir for positive cultures or onset of symptoms (if positive, requires lumbar puncture)
- Cesarean section, primary or recurrent infection with rupture of membranes less than 4 hours: Surface cultures at 24 to 48 hours, observe, treat if positive cultures or onset of symptoms
- History of genital HSV without lesions at birth: Observe

■ **Complications**

- Skin/eye/mucous membranes disease: Low risk of morbidity and mortality
- CNS disease: 5% mortality but 60% of survivors have severe neurologic sequelae
- Disseminated disease: 30% mortality but fewer than 20% of survivors have neurologic sequelae

18 Fever

Elizabeth R. Alpern, MD, MSCE and Samir S. Shah, MD

Febrile Neonate

- Fever (38.0°C or higher) in a well-appearing infant (0 to 60 days of age) without identifiable source of infection. Infant is at risk for occult serious bacterial infections (SBI)

■ Epidemiology

- Epidemiology, evaluation, and treatment are differentiated by age (0 to 28 days and 29 to 60 days of life) due to stratified risk of SBI and sensitivity of screening procedure
- 10% to 15% of neonates with fever have SBI

■ Risk Factors

- Untreated pre- or perinatal maternal infection (e.g., *Neisseria gonorrhoeae*)
- Exposure to pathogens from birth canal or postnatal exposure to ill contacts
- Relative immune compromised state of young infants

■ Etiology

- Most common pathogens: *Escherichia coli*, *Klebsiella* species, *Streptococcus pneumoniae*, group B *Streptococcus*, *Staphylococcus aureus*, *Enterococcus* spp., *Listeria monocytogenes*

■ History/Physical Examination

- Vague or nonspecific signs and symptoms of illness (may present with just an isolated fever)
- Fever, irritability, lethargy, poor feeding, emesis, diarrhea, jaundice, rash
- Search for findings that suggest a likely cause (see "Differential Diagnosis")
- Lack of ill appearance does not rule out SBI in neonates

■ Additional Studies

- *Negative screen* (Philadelphia protocol) indicates low risk for SBI (Baker et al):

- Well appearance and normal physical exam
- WBC count 5000 to 15,000/mm^3
- Band/neutrophil ratio: Less than 0.2
- Enhanced (unspun) urinalysis (UA) less than 10 cells/mm^3 and negative Gram stain or no leukocyte esterate/nitrites by dipstick and less than 5 wbc/hpf by microscopy
- Lumbar puncture (LP) less than 8 cells/mm^3 and negative Gram stain
- Normal CXR, stool smear without WBCs (perform if specific signs)
- *Positive screen* (higher risk for SBI) if *any one or more* of above criteria not met

■ Differential Diagnosis

- Abscess, cellulitis, bacteremia, bacterial meningitis, bacterial enteritis, pneumonia, septic arthritis, osteomyelitis, urinary tract infection, aseptic meningitis, HSV encephalitis, bronchiolitis, and nonbacterial gastroenteritis

■ Management

- Criteria: Age 0 to 60 days and fever greater than 38.0°C without identifiable source
- Evaluation: CBC, UA, and blood, urine, and CSF cultures. Consider CXR if hypoxia or respiratory findings. Consider stool culture if diarrhea
- Specific Management:
  - Age 0 to 28 days: All infants require admission and IV ampicillin and gentamicin or cefotaxime while awaiting culture results
  - Age 29 to 60 days: "Negative screen" permits discharge without antibiotics. Reevaluate in 24 hours
  - Age 29 to 60 days: "Positive screen" requires admission and IV ampicillin and gentamicin or cefotaxime while awaiting culture results

■ Complications

- If SBI diagnosed then complications related to disease process (e.g., hearing loss with meningitis, renal scarring with pyelonephritis)

Febrile Infant

- Occult bacteremia (OB) is the presence of pathogenic bacteria in the blood of a healthy, well-appearing, febrile (T > 39.0°C) child without a focal bacterial source of infection. Important because of risk of progression to focal infection (e.g., meningitis)

■ Epidemiology/Risk Factors

- Traditional risk group is aged 2 to 24 months (some studies show up to 36 months)
- OB occurs in less than 2% of febrile children 2 to 24 months of age immunized with *Haemophilus influenzae* type B (HIB) vaccine
- Risk of OB is higher with a WBC count greater than 15,000/mm^3

■ Etiology

- Common: *S. pneumoniae*
- Uncommon: *Salmonella* spp., group A *Streptococcus*, *Moraxella catarrhalis*
- *H. influenzae* type B rare since introduction of HIB vaccine
- Rate of *S. pneumoniae* infection may be lowered by conjugate vaccines

■ History/Physical Examination

- Determine risk factors (age, immunization status)
- Assess for findings that exclude patient from OB diagnosis: 1) Underlying condition (e.g., primary immune deficiency, sickle cell); 2) focal bacterial infection (e.g., meningitis, osteomyelitis, pneumonia)

■ Additional Studies

- Consider other studies to determine focal infection (e.g., urine culture, CXR)
- Blood culture is diagnostic but contamination rate is 2%
- White blood count or C-reactive protein used by some to identify those at higher risk

■ Management

- Careful exam and follow-up are mandatory in all patients
- Some experts advocate blood culture
- Other experts also recommend presumptive antibiotics (IM ceftriaxone) in those at highest risk (white blood counts 15,000/mm^3 and higher) in hopes of reducing serious sequelae in those ultimately found to have OB

■ Complications

- Focal infection including cellulitis, meningitis, pneumonia, and osteomyelitis

Fever of Unknown Origin

- Fever of unknown origin (FUO) indicates 1) prolonged fever (more than 2 weeks); 2) documented temperature greater than 38.3°C on multiple occasions; and 3) uncertain cause

■ Epidemiology/Risk Factors

- 50% of patients referred for FUO evaluation have multiple, unrelated, self-limited infections; misinterpretation of normal temperature variation; or absence of fever

■ Etiology

- 40% to 60% of children have resolution of fever without a specific diagnosis.
- Infectious causes:
  - Common: Sinopulmonary infections; systemic viral syndrome; UTI; meningitis; enteric infection (e.g., *Salmonella, Yersinia, Campylobacter*); osteomyelitis.
  - Less common: Tuberculosis; cat-scratch disease; infectious mononucleosis; Lyme disease; Rocky Mountain spotted fever; ehrlichiosis; malaria; dental abscess; brain abscess; endocarditis; HIV
  - Rare: Q fever, brucellosis, tularemia, leptospirosis; parvovirus B19; histoplasmosis; blastomycosis; coccidioidomycosis, syphilis

■ Pathogenesis

- Temperature normally varies with peak in early evening and nadir in early morning

■ History/Physical Examination

- Exposure to animals: Includes rodents and farm animals; unpasteurized milk; and household contacts with occupational exposure
- Tick or flea bites (e.g., tularemia, brucellosis, Lyme)
- Travel history: Includes prophylactic measures (e.g., malaria prophylaxis) and close contacts who have traveled
- Medications, antecedent illness or trauma, family history (e.g., immune deficiency)
- Search for findings that suggest a likely cause (see "Etiology" and "Differential Diagnosis")
- Check growth parameters, skin findings, bone tenderness, gait and muscle mass

■ Additional Studies

- See Table 18-1 for suggested evaluation. Not every patient needs every test

■ Differential Diagnosis

- Noninfectious causes: Systemic juvenile rheumatoid arthritis (JRA); systemic lupus erythematosus; sarcoidosis; vasculitis; malignancy; Kawasaki; inflammatory bowel disease; drug or central fever; periodic fever syndrome; factitious fever

■ TABLE 18-1 Tests to Consider in Evaluation of Fever of Unknown Origin

	Initial	Subsequent
Blood	Blood culture CRP, ESR Liver function tests HIV testing Initial serologies[a]	Repeat blood culture Second-line serologies[b]
Urine	UA and culture	N/A
Stool	Hemoccult testing Culture (bacterial/viral) Ova/parasite testing	C. difficile toxins A and B
Radiologic	CXR	Sinus CT Upper GI barium study Abdominal ultrasound MRI of pelvis, spine, or other Bone or gallium scan Echocardiogram
Miscellaneous	Tuberculin skin test Nasal aspirate for rapid viral antigen detection Throat culture	Ophthalmologic examination LP Bone marrow biopsy Evaluate for immune deficiency (see Chapter 22)

[a] Initial serologies: EBV, CMV, streptococcal enzymes, antinuclear antibodies.
[b] Second-line serologies: Hepatitis A, B, C, tularemia, brucellosis, leptospirosis, Rocky Mountain spotted fever, ehrlichiosis, Q fever (if relevant exposures).
Adapted from Calello DP, Shah SS. The child with fever of unknown origin. *Pediatr Case Rev* 2002;2:226–239.

■ **Management**
- Careful and repeated history and physical may reveal diagnosis. "Shotgun" approach to evaluation rarely useful but certain initial studies (Table 18-1) may provide insight

■ **Complications**
- Related to cause of FUO; iatrogenic complications during overzealous evaluation

Periodic Fever Syndromes

- Recurrent fevers that last from a few days to a few weeks, separated by symptom-free intervals of variable duration

■ **Epidemiology/Etiology (Table 18-2)**

- PFAPA (periodic fever, aphthous stomatitis, pharyngitis, and cervical adenitis) is most common periodic fever syndrome. Most recurrent fevers *not* due to a periodic fever syndrome

■ **History/Physical Examination (Table 18-2)**

- Distinguish recurrent fever with regular as opposed to unpredictable intervals

■ **TABLE 18-2 Features of Some Periodic Fever Syndromes**

	PFAPA	FMF[c]	Hyper-IgD	TRAPS
Epidemiology	None	Armenian, Arab, Turkish, Sephardic Jews	Dutch, French	Irish, Scottish
Typical age of onset	2–3 yr	<20 yr[a]	<1 yr	<20 yr
Duration of episode	4–5 d	1–2 d	3–7 d	>7 d
Frequency of recurrence	21–42 d	7–28 d[b]	14–28 d[b]	None
Symptoms other than fever	Stomatitis, pharyngitis, adenitis	Peritonitis monoarthritis, other serositis, erysipelas-like skin lesions (40%)	Cervical adenopathy, abdominal pain, diarrhea	Arthralgias, myalgias, conjunctivitis, abdominal pain, erythematous macules, edematous plaques
Laboratory findings	Nonspecific	Low C5a inhibitor in serosal fluids	Serum IgD >100 IU/mL; elevated IgA (80%)	Low serum type 1 TNF receptor
Therapy	Single-dose prednisone at symptom onset; prophylactic cimetidine	Colchicine (daily)	None	Corticosteroids; etanercept (binds TNF-α)

[a] Onset younger than 10 years in 50%.
[b] Often unpredictable.
[c] FAF, familial mediterranean fever

Adapted from Drenth JPH, van Der Meer JWM. Hereditary periodic fever. *N Engl J Med* 2001;345:1748–1757.

■ **Additional Studies (Table 18-2)**

- CBC with differential twice per week for 2 months to exclude cyclic neutropenia
- Mutation screening helpful in some situations: MEFV gene (70% with FMF); V377I mutation (hyper-IgD); type 1 TNF receptor (TRAPS)

■ **Differential Diagnosis**

- Infectious: Repeated viral infections; Epstein-Barr virus; parvovirus B19; recurrent UTI; brucellosis; tuberculosis; relapsing malaria; chronic meningococcemia
- Immunologic/inflammatory: Crohn disease; systemic JRA; Behçet disease; familial cold urticaria; Muckle-Wells syndrome
- Other: Cyclic neutropenia; lymphoma; leukemia; central fever; drug fever.

■ **Management**

See Table 18-2.

■ **Complications**

- PFAPA: Resolves within 5 years of onset in 40%; no long-term sequelae known
- FMF: Amyloid deposition in kidneys, spleen, liver, heart, and other organs. Colchicine arrests amyloidosis and reverses proteinuria
- Hyper-IgD: Attacks diminish with age.
- TRAPS: Amyloid deposition in kidneys (25%) leads to renal impairment

Fever in the Returning Traveler

■ **Epidemiology**

- More than 20% of travelers report illness associated with travel
- 3% of international travelers are affected by fevers; malaria is most common cause

■ **Risk Factors**

- Increased risk with visits to family/friends or "adventure" tours

■ **Etiology/Pathogenesis**

See Table 18-3.

■ **TABLE 18-3 Causes of Fever in the Returning Traveler**

Organism or disease	Transmission	Incubation	Associated Symptoms
Malaria	Mosquito	Days to years	CNS findings; myalgias; GI findings; jaundice; HSM
Dengue	Mosquito	< 14 d	Headache; myalgias; adenopathy; rash; splenomegaly
Rickettsia	Tick or mite	< 14 d	Headache, myalgia
Bacterial enteritis	Contaminated food/water	< 14 d	Undifferentiated fever
Leptospirosis	Animal urine; Contaminated water/soil	< 14 d to 6 wk	Headache; myalgias; hemorrhage; conjunctival suffusion; jaundice
Typhoid fever	Contaminated food/water	< 14 d to 6 wk	CNS findings
Trypanosomiasis	Tsetse fly	< 14 d	CNS findings; splenomegaly
Viral hemorrhagic fever (see Chapter 24)	Mosquito; direct/airborne	< 21 d	Hemorrhage; jaundice; splenomegaly
Influenza	Direct/airborne	< 14 d	Respiratory findings
Hepatitis A or E	Contaminated food/water	14 d to 6 wk	Jaundice; hepatomegaly
Schistosomiasis	Cercariae in fresh water	4–8 wk	Headache; myalgias; arthralgias; cough; diarrhea; HSM
Q fever	Inhalation of animal source	14 d to 6 wk	Respiratory findings
Tuberculosis	Inhalation	Weeks to months	Respiratory findings
Hepatitis B	Sexual transmission	Weeks to months	Jaundice; hepatomegaly
HIV	Sexual transmission	Weeks to months	Headache; myalgias; arthralgias; adenopathy; sore throat; diarrhea; mucocutaneous lesions

■ **History/Physical Examination (Table 18-3)**

• Travel history; exposure history (animal exposure, freshwater swimming, mosquito bites, raw or undercooked foods, untreated drinking water, sexual encounters)

- Duration of fever; departure and return dates to calculate potential incubation period
- Immunizations; antimalarial chemoprophylaxis

■ Additional Studies

- Determine tests as indicated by history, physical examination, time course of illness
- Consider: Peripheral blood for malaria, CBC, liver function tests, urinalysis, blood culture, stool culture and ova/parasite examination, CXR, tuberculin skin test
- Specific serologic assays: Dengue virus, rickettsiae, schistosomes, leptospira, HIV

■ Differential Diagnosis

- Infections unrelated to specific travel itinerary (e.g., sinusitis)

■ Management

- Management options must be tailored to specific disease process
- Test for malaria in all patients returning from malaria endemic area with fever

Kawasaki Syndrome

- Small- and medium-vessel vasculitis (also termed mucocutaneous lymph node syndrome)

■ Epidemiology

- Median age, 2 years; 80% of patients younger than 5 years; only 5% older than 10 years
- Incomplete (atypical) presentation more common in those younger than 12 months

■ Risk Factors/Etiology

- Incidence in Japanese > blacks > whites; in United States, occurs in 10 per 100,000 children. Rate is 10-fold higher in Japan. Cause unknown

■ Pathogenesis

- Unknown precipitant causes perivascular infiltration by macrophages, monocytes, lymphocytes, and others. Inflammation disrupts vessel wall, leading to aneurysms

■ **History/Physical Examination**

- Diagnostic criteria include (fever) lasting 5 or more days plus at least four of the following:
  - Bilateral nonpurulent conjunctivitis: Limbic sparing, bulbar > palpebral involvement
  - Oral changes: Lips dry, cracked, bleeding, and peeling; strawberry tongue
  - Cervical adenopathy: Greater than 1.5 cm; usually unilateral; absent in 50%
  - Extremity changes: Palmar erythema; swollen hands/feet; desquamation (2 to 3 weeks)
  - Polymorphous rash: Usually begins 3 to 5 days after fever; classically at groin/buttocks
- Associated features: Aseptic meningitis (25% to 40% of patients undergoing LP); uveitis (80%); acute myocarditis (30%); diarrhea (25% to 50%); gallbladder hydrops (10%); hepatitis (50%); pancreatitis; urethritis (50%); arthralgias/arthritis (33%)
- Incomplete or atypical Kawasaki cases do not fulfill above criteria but still may develop coronary aneurysms

■ **Additional Studies**

- WBC count: 95% more than $10,000/mm^3$; 50% more than $15,000/mm^3$
- Hemoglobin: 75% less than two standard deviations below the mean
- Platelets: Increase during second week; usually increase to more than $750,000/mm^3$
- ESR: Elevated in more than 90%
- Urinalysis: Sterile pyuria due to urethritis may be missed by bladder catheterization; therefore, fresh void specimen preferred.
- Echocardiogram: Detects coronary aneurysms; usually present at 10 to 21 days

■ **Differential Diagnosis**

- Infectious: Measles; scarlet fever; Epstein-Barr virus; adenovirus; enterovirus; parvovirus B19; *S. aureus* toxin–mediated disease; Rocky Mountain spotted fever
- Allergic/rheumatologic: Drug reaction; Stevens-Johnson syndrome; systemic JRA; polyarteritis nodosum; Reiter syndrome

■ **Management**

- Intravenous immune globulin (IVIG): 2 g/kg over 12 hours. Repeat if still febrile 24 hours after completion of first dose (10% of patients)

- - IVIG within 10 days of onset reduces coronary aneurysm risk from 15%–25% to 5%.
- Aspirin for anti-inflammatory and antiplatelet effect
  - Initially high-dose (80–100 mg/kg/d divided into four doses)
  - When afebrile use 3–5 mg/kg daily; continue until platelet count normal (usually 6 to 8 weeks); dipyridamole for aspirin-allergic patients
- Corticosteroid therapy controversial but under study
- Repeat echocardiogram 2 weeks after diagnosis and 1 month later
  - Detection of aneurysm requires continued cardiology follow-up

■ Complications

- Coronary artery aneurysms: Small (less than 8 mm) aneurysms regress; larger ones often persist and may rupture or develop stenosis or thrombosis; overall mortality less than 0.3%

19 Fever and Rash

Louis M. Bell, MD

Fever and Petechiae

- Petechiae, caused by extravasation of red blood cells, are non-blanching erythematous macular skin lesions 1 mm or greater in size
- Febrile infants and children with a petechial rash raise the concern of invasive bacterial infection caused by *Neisseria meningitidis* or other organisms

■ Epidemiology

- 2% to 20% of children with fever and petechiae have invasive infection; risk highest if under 2 years old or ill appearing

■ Etiology

- Bacterial: *N. meningitidis, Streptococcus pneumoniae, Haemophilus influenzae* type B, *Escherichia coli*
- Viral: Influenza, parainfluenza, enteroviruses, Epstein-Barr virus (EBV), dengue, adenovirus, respiratory syncytial virus, rotavirus
- Other infections: Rocky Mountain spotted fever (RMSF), ehrlichiosis, scarlet fever

■ Differential Diagnosis

- Drug eruption, acute leukemia, subacute bacterial endocarditis, cough/emesis

■ History/Physical Examination

- Close exposure to someone with meningococcemia
- Serious findings include fever, headache, severely ill appearing, mental status changes, signs of compensated shock (unexplained tachycardia, widened pulse pressure, bounding pulses)
- Important considerations: What is the distribution? Is the rash along the course of the superior vena cava secondary to vomiting or cough? Did the petechiae occur after tourniquet application? Is there evidence of pharyngitis or scarlet fever with petechiae only above the nipple line?

■ TABLE 19-1 Suggested Management for Children with Fever and Petechiae

Suggested Management		Signs/Symptoms/Lab Data
Admit to the ICU, stabilize with fluids, antibiotics, vasopressors	IF	Purpura, shock, sepsis, hemorrhage
Admission and IV antibiotics after complete sepsis evaluation	IF	Less than 6–12 mo of age, ill-appearing or immunocompromised
Discharge to home with follow-up in 24 h on antistreptococcal antibiotic if appropriate	IF	Well appearing with cough or emesis and petechiae above nipple line and positive streptococcal antigen test
Discharge with follow-up in 12 to 24 h. Presumptive antibiotic therapy (IM ceftriaxone)	IF	Normal WBC, band count less than 500/mm^3, ANC 1500–9000/mm^3, normal PT, and no progression of rash
Admission with completion of lumbar puncture and intravenous fluids/antibiotics	IF	Any abnormal laboratory data (as above) or progression of rash

■ Additional Studies

- Well-appearing children with petechiae and normal WBC count, band count, and prothrombin time are at lower risk for invasive disease

■ Management (Table 19-1)

- No consensus on management of well-appearing children with fever and petechiae

Rickettsial Infections

- Rickettsial infections are categorized as follows:
  - Spotted fever group: Rickettsial pox (*Rickettsia akari*); scrub typhus (*Rickettsia* and tsutsugamushi); Rocky Mountain spotted fever (*Rickettsia rickettsii*)
  - Typhus group: Endemic typhus (*Rickettsia typhi*) (murine or flea-borne typhus); epidemic typhus (*Rickettsia prowazekii*) (louse-borne typhus)
  - Miscellaneous: Ehrlichiosis (*Ehrlichia* species); Q fever (*Coxiella burnetii*)
- Discussion below focuses on RMSF and ehrlichiosis

■ Epidemiology

- Most RMSF infections are in South Atlantic coastal, western, and south central states

- RMSF usually occurs from April to September, ehrlichiosis from May to July

■ Risk Factors

- Exposure to arthropod vectors: Ticks, mites, fleas
- Exposure to dogs, wild rodents, rabbits, and opossums

■ Pathogenesis

- Rickettsiae are obligate intracellular pathogens. Humans are incidental host
- Systemic capillary and small vessel endothelial damage results in vasculitis and shock

■ History/Physical Examination

- Suspect rickettsial infections in those with flulike illness in spring or summer
- High fever, severe frontal headache, malaise, myalgias, and vomiting
- Rash appears 2 to 3 days (range 1 to 14 days) after the onset of illness; more likely with RMSF than with ehrlichia
- Rash starts on the wrists and ankles and then the palms and soles, face, and trunk. It progresses from macular to papular to petechial to purpuric
- Hepatomegaly, meningismus, decreased breath sounds with rales
- A necrotic eschar ("tache noir" or "black spot"; 30% to 90% of patients) originates at the site of the bite. Look for this in the scalp with associated regional lymphadenopathy

■ Additional Studies

- Leukopenia, thrombocytopenia, elevated serum hepatic transaminases, hyponatremia
- Fourfold rise in specific acute and convalescent antibodies by indirect fluorescent antibody assay (sensitivity greater than 90%). Antibodies detectable 7 to 14 days after onset
- Ehrlichiosis: Light microscopy of blood smear reveals morulae in neutrophil cytoplasm (50% of cases)
- RMSF: If rash present, immunofluorescence or immunoperoxidase staining of skin biopsy reveals *R. rickettsii* in vascular endothelium (sensitivity 70% to 90%)
- Polymerase chain reaction (PCR) assay available in some research settings

■ Differential Diagnosis

- Measles; meningococcemia; secondary syphilis; viral infections (especially enteroviruses); infectious mononucleosis

■ Management
- Early suspicion and prompt therapy is vital to a good outcome
- Treat with **doxycycline** or tetracycline for 5 to 7 days. Limited data on alternate agents: In patients allergic to tetracycline class, consider rifampin or fluoroquinolones for ehrlichiosis and chloramphenicol or fluoroquinolones for RMSF.

■ Complications
- Venous thrombosis; pneumonitis; pericarditis; myocarditis; pleural effusions

Lyme Disease

■ Epidemiology
- The most common vector-borne disease in the United States
- Most cases occur in the Northeast (Maine to Maryland), the upper Midwest (Wisconsin and Minnesota), and the West (California and Oregon).
- Most cases in June, July, and August. Peak incidence is at age 5 to 14 years

■ Risk Factors
- *Borrelia burgdorferi* lives in tick midgut so infection requires more than 24 to 36 hours of attachment
- Environment risk: Region, climate, landscape, and close association with wildlife
- Behavioral risk: Woodcutting, outdoor activities (more than 30 hours per week)

■ Etiology
- Lyme disease caused by the spirochete *B. burgdorferi* and transmitted by *Ixodes* ticks

■ Pathogenesis
- Stage 1: Localized erythema migrans (EM) rash. After the bite, the *B. burgdorferi* organisms spread superficially through the skin and tissue
- Stage 2: Early dissemination follows stage 1 within days or weeks; may result in multiple skin lesions (disseminated EM) or affect the joints, nervous system, or heart
- Stage 3: Late dissemination (affects joints) follows stage 1 within weeks or months.

■ History
- History of rash with a slowly expanding skin lesion (EM)

- The skin lesion may be accompanied by a history of flulike symptoms (malaise, fatigue, headache, arthralgias, myalgias, fever, regional lymphadenopathy)

■ Physical Examination

Stage 1
- Rash of **EM** (more than 5 cm in diameter)
- Usually macular, but may be slightly raised with occasional central ulceration

Stage 2
- Neurologic: Lymphocytic meningitis; subtle encephalitis; **cranial neuropathies** (unilateral or bilateral, especially 7th); optic nerve involvement leading to blindness (more common in children); motor or sensory radiculoneuritis; cerebellar ataxia
- Cardiac: Commonly **atrioventricular block**; occasionally acute myopericarditis; rarely cardiomegaly or pancarditis
  - Occurs in 5% of untreated patients
- Joint involvement: Arthritis (knee most commonly)

Stage 3
- Prolonged neurologic abnormalities including motor or sensory radiculoneuritis, cerebellar ataxia, subacute encephalopathy, memory impairment, sleep disturbances

■ Additional Studies

- Base decision for serologic testing on finding the above signs and symptoms
- If EM is found, no laboratory testing needed
- Antibody testing: Initial testing by ELISA to *B. burgdorferi*. If IgM or IgG positive, confirm by Western blotting. ELISA alone has high false-positive rate
- PCR of joint fluid (usually not needed) for diagnosis of Lyme arthritis
- CSF antibodies may be diagnostic of Lyme meningitis. CSF PCR test has poor sensitivity

■ Differential Diagnosis

- EM-like rash: Tinea corporis, insect bite, eczema, cellulitis, erythema multiforme
- Rash and arthritis: Serum sickness, juvenile rheumatoid arthritis, acute rheumatic fever, systemic lupus erythematosus
- Meningitis/neurologic abnormalities: See Chapter 7

■ Management

- *Stage 1*-EM: Older than 8 years, **doxycycline**; 8 years or younger (or pregnancy), **amoxicillin**

- Treat for 14 to 21 days. Alternate for allergy use cefuroxime or macrolide
- *Stages 2 and 3*
  - Disseminated EM or isolated Bell palsy: Same as for stage 1
  - Arthritis: Same as for stage 1 but treat for 28 days. Some require ceftriaxone
  - Meningitis, other neurologic involvement, or carditis: **Ceftriaxone** for 21 to 28 days
- First recurrence of arthritis may result from incomplete initial treatment and warrants second course of antibiotics. Subsequent recurrences treated with NSAIDs. Recurrences diminish in frequency over 1 year

■ Complications
- Untreated localized disease may progress to early or late dissemination

Major Childhood Viral Exanthems

- Major childhood exanthems cause systemic illness and a characteristic rash
- Exanthems: Blanching macular or papular lesions (less than 1 cm in diameter)
- Morbilliform: Lesions that coalesce (e.g., measles)
- Scarlatiniform: Lesions with a sandpaper feel on palpation (e.g., scarlet fever)

■ Etiology
- Enteroviruses are most common cause (Table 19-2)
- Bacterial causes include group A *Streptococcus, Staphylococcus aureus,* and *Arcanobacterium haemolyticum*

■ Pathogenesis
- Most commonly either 1) infection of the dermal blood vessel endothelium (e.g., measles) or 2) host immunologic reaction against the pathogen (e.g., parvovirus B19)
- Circulating toxins cause the scarlatiniform exanthem in *S. pyogenes* and *S. aureus*

■ History/Physical Examination (Table 19-2)
- Exposure to person with similar illness or pets/animals; recent travel; immunizations
- Elicit prodromal symptoms and where rash started and pattern of spread

■ TABLE 19-2 Recognizable Childhood Exanthems: Patterns of Progression and Distribution

Disease	Rash Progression	Distribution/ Characteristics	Etiology
Measles	Koplik spots; nape of the neck to trunk	Morbilliform trunk and face less on extremities	Measles virus
Fifth disease (erythema infectiosum)	Slapped cheeks to trunk	Macular, fades and reappears with temperature change mainly on trunk	Parvovirus B19
Papular purpuric gloves and socks syndrome	Papular to petechial to purpura of hands/ wrist/ankles/feet	Purpura of hand/ feet edema	Parvovirus B19
Pityriasis rosea	Herald patch (less than 1 cm) neck and trunk	Papular with scale on trunk, upper arms	Viral suspected (HHV-6 or 7)
Unilateral laterothoracic exanthem of childhood	Remains unilateral in groin or axilla with spread to unilateral trunk	1-mm papules to coalesced eczematous patches	Viral (?)
Gianotti-Crosti (papular acrodermatitis)	Cheeks, extensor sides of extremities to buttocks	Papular, pink, flat-topped spares trunk, indues face and extremities	EBV, CMV, HBV
Scarlet fever	Neck to trunk and extremities, intense rash creases elbows, axillae, groin	Fine papular (sandpaper) erythema of skin, face spared. Desquamation after 5–7 d	Group A Streptococcus
Roseola infantum	After fever resolves, rash on trunk to neck, face and extremities	2- to 5-mm pink papules rash fades in 1–3 d	HHV-6 HHV-7

■ Additional Studies

- In well-appearing children with fever and exanthema, a careful history and examination often leads to the correct diagnosis without the need for further studies
- Measles: Serology, measles-specific IgM
- Rubella: Serology, rubella-specific IgM; culture from nasal specimen
- Human herpes virus 6 (HHV-6): Testing not available, commercial antibody and PCR reaction assays in development
- Parvovirus B19: Serology, parvovirus-specific IgM; PCR in immunocompromised

- EBV: Serology, EBV-specific antibody profile; PCR in immuno-compromised
- Enteroviruses: Culture blood/urine early; PCR blood, urine, CSF
- Adenovirus: Culture and rapid antigen detection on secretions; PCR blood/urine

■ Management

- Most childhood exanthems are benign and self-limited, and resolve within several days
- For streptococcal pharyngitis, **penicillin or amoxicillin** for 10 days (see Chapter 8).

20 Infections in Children with Cancer

Anne F. Reilly, MD, MPH

Fever and Neutropenia

- Fever in a child with cancer may be the first sign of serious invasive infection
- Fever: Temperature greater than 38.3°C even once, or 38.0°C or higher for more than 1 hour
- Neutropenia: Absolute neutrophil count (ANC) less than 500/mm³, or less than 1000 mm³ and falling

■ Epidemiology

- A definite source of infection is found in 20% to 40% of febrile neutropenic patients

■ Risk Factors

- Low risk of serious infection: 1) ANC 100 cells/mm³ or more; 2) neutropenia expected to last less than 10 days; 3) normal CXR; 4) no other significant comorbidities
- High risk of serious infection: All patients not at low risk

■ Etiology

- Infectious:
  - **Bacteria**:
    - Gram positive (most common): Coagulase-negative staphylococci, *Staphylococcus aureus*, viridans streptococci, enterococci, *Clostridium difficile*
    - Gram negative: *Escherichia coli*, *Klebsiella*, *Enterobacter*, *Pseudomonas* spp., anaerobes
  - **Fungi**: *Candida* spp., *Aspergillus* spp., *Pneumocystis carinii*, cryptococci
  - **Viruses**: Herpes simplex virus (HSV), varicella-zoster virus (VZV), cytomegalovirus (CMV), Epstein-Barr virus (EBV), respiratory syncytial virus (RSV), adenovirus, influenza virus, parainfluenza virus
- Noninfectious: Medications; underlying malignancy; blood products

■ Pathogenesis

- Disruption of skin/mucous membranes 2° to therapy, surgery, indwelling catheters
- Depletion of host defense cells (neutrophils, lymphocytes, others)

■ History/Physical Examination

- Recent chemotherapy (to judge expected period of neutropenia)
- Any complaint could be important: Cough, headache, diarrhea, dysuria, rash
- Infection may not be obvious when the ANC is low; neutrophils are critical to the inflammatory response. Tenderness may be the only localizing sign of infection
- Careful examination of entire body; examine skin for rashes, ulcers, vesicles, erythema

■ Additional Studies

- CBC, chemistries, urinalysis (may not see pyuria in a neutropenic patient)
- Blood cultures, including samples from each lumen of a central venous catheter
- Other cultures as indicated: Urine, stool, CSF, oral or skin lesions
- CXR: Consider in all patients, particularly with respiratory symptoms

■ Differential Diagnosis

- Common sites of infection in febrile neutropenic patients include bloodstream; skin/soft tissue; mouth/oropharynx; gastrointestinal (GI) tract; lungs; sinuses

■ Management

- **Antibiotics**: Prompt empiric broad-spectrum antimicrobial therapy

Potential Regimens

Potential regimens may vary depending on institution:

- Monotherapy: Ceftazidime or cefepime or carbapenems (imipenem/cilastatin, meropenem)
- Duotherapy: Aminoglycoside (gentamicin, tobramycin, or amikacin) *plus* ticarcillin-clavulanic acid or piperacillin-tazobactam or cefepime or ceftazidime or carbapenem
- *Add* **vancomycin** when resistant organisms are common, particularly viridans group streptococci. Vancomycin can be discontinued after 24 to 48 hours if no such organism is found on culture

- Specific clinical events (e.g., perianal cellulitis, breakthrough bacteremia) may require modification of therapy

Continuation of Therapy
- Afebrile by days 3 to 5
  - When ANC is greater than 500 cells/mm³ for 2 days, stop antibiotics
  - If ANC is less than 500 cells/mm³: If low risk, continue IV antibiotics or consider change to oral antibiotics (ciprofloxacin + amoxicillin-clavulanate as inpatient). If high risk, continue IV antibiotics. Some centers consider stopping antibiotics if ANC is greater than 100/mm³ and increasing
- Persistent fever without clear etiology
  - If low risk for fungal infection, continue antibiotics until ANC begins rising
  - If high risk for fungal infection, fever lasting more than 5 to 7 days, and neutropenia resolution not imminent, start presumptive antifungal therapy (First line: amphotericin B preparation; alternative: voriconazole)

Adjuncts to Therapy
- Antiviral drugs when appropriate: 1) **Acyclovir** (HSV or VZV); 2) **ribavirin** (RSV); 3) **amantadine, oseltamivir**, or others (influenza virus)
- Granulocyte transfusions and colony-stimulating factors are not routinely recommended. May be used in neutropenic patients with severe fungal infection, or uncontrolled bacterial infection despite appropriate antibiotic therapy

Skin Infections

■ Etiology (Table 20-1)/Pathogenesis
- Common skin flora gain access to skin via breaks caused by catheters, wounds, and chemotherapy-induced lesions such as oral ulcers
- Immunosuppression caused by therapy, such as neutropenia, and decreased T-cell response, allows organisms to cause infection

■ History/Physical Examination
- Rash quality and location; history of trauma; recent procedures; fever, muscle aches, jaundice
- Skin and mucous membranes; note vesicles, papules, necrosis, discoloration
- Vascular access catheters: Erythema or tenderness over the tunnel indicates tunnel infection; pus or erythema within 2 cm of exit site indicates an exit site infection

■ TABLE 20-1 Causes and Manifestations of Skin Infections in Children with Cancer

	Common Organisms	Typical Skin Manifestations
Bacteria	Staphylococcus aureus	Impetigo, cellulitis, folliculitis
	Streptococcus pyogenes	Impetigo, cellulitis, folliculitis
	Nocardia	Nodules, abscesses, cellulitis
	Mycobacterium tuberculosis	Nodules, lymphangitis
	Nontuberculous mycobacteria	Papules, nodules, ulcers
	Pseudomonas aeruginosa	Cellulitis, pyoderma, ecthyma gangrenosum
Fungi	Dermatophytes (e.g., Microsporum)	Tinea pedis, tinea capitis, nail infections
	Candida spp.	Oral thrush, dermatitis, nodules with systemic infection
	Histoplasma capsulatum	Rash (macules, papules, plaques)
	Aspergillus	Ulcer with eschar (often at IV sites)
Viruses	Human papillomavirus	Warts
	Varicella-zoster virus	Shingles, chickenpox
	Herpes simplex virus	Gingivostomatitis, keratitis, genital infections

■ Additional Studies

- Aspirate or biopsy of representative lesions, with culture and pathology if possible
- Vesicles scraped at base for direct fluorescent antibody testing for VZV or HSV
- Blood cultures when fever present; chemistries for hepatic or renal involvement

■ Management

- Systemic antimicrobial therapy appropriate to the infecting organism indicated. Treat intravenously if significant immuno-suppression or neutropenia present
- VZV infection should be managed with intravenous acyclovir; systemic disease can develop quickly and can be life-threatening
- Local therapies include drainage of abscesses, excision of necrotic or nonviable tissue. Management of tunnel infections includes catheter removal

Pulmonary Infections

■ Epidemiology

- Respiratory infections are among the most common infections in cancer patients

- Up to 10% of fever/neutropenia episodes may be caused by pneumonia

■ Risk Factors
- Those with leukemia, lymphoma, and stem cell transplant are at particularly high risk for pulmonary bacterial and fungal disease
- Graft versus host disease, steroid therapy, radiation therapy to lungs increase risk

■ Etiology
- Localized infiltrates:
  - Bacteria: Respiratory pathogens, *Mycobacteria, Legionella, Nocardia*
  - Fungus: *Aspergillus, Fusarium* spp., *Pseudallescheria boydii, Rhizopus, Mucor, Candida*
  - Viral: HSV, VZV—less likely
  - *Mycoplasma pneumoniae*
- Diffuse infiltrates:
  - Bacteria: Usual respiratory pathogens, gram positive and negative
  - Fungus: Most common is *P. carinii*
  - Viral: Cytomegalovirus (CMV), RSV, adenovirus, HSV, VZV, influenza virus, parainfluenza virus, human herpes virus 6 (HHV-6)
  - *Mycoplasma pneumoniae*

■ Pathogenesis
- Colonization of the upper respiratory tract provides a close reservoir of pathogens
- Immunosuppression, poor mucociliary function lead to decreased pathogen clearance

■ History/Physical Examination
- Fever, chest pain, cough, dyspnea, hypoxemia
- Evaluate work of breathing: Retractions, tachypnea
- Auscultation of the chest: Rales, rhonchi, wheezing, rubs, decreased breath sounds
- Dullness to percussion, egophony

■ Additional Studies
- Blood work: Blood counts, blood cultures, arterial blood gas in very sick patients
- Sputum collection, nasopharyngeal (NP) aspirates for viral antigen testing and culture, consider *Mycoplasma* polymerase chain reaction of NP aspirate

- CXR; CT scans for further evaluation, or if CXR negative with an abnormal lung examination
- If patient is progressing or very ill, consider bronchoalveolar lavage (BAL) or lung biopsy (open biopsy or transthoracic needle biopsy) for pathology and cultures

■ Differential Diagnosis

- Drug-induced or chemical pneumonitis; hemorrhage; atelectasis; pulmonary edema; tumor; lymphoma; leukemic infiltrates; radiation pneumonitis

■ Management

- **Local infiltrate:**
  - Initial therapy with broad-spectrum antibiotics (see "Management" under "Fever and Neutropenia"). Consider adding macrolide if *Mycoplasma* or *Legionella* suspected
  - If no improvement in 3 or 4 days, obtain tissue diagnosis if possible with BAL, or biopsy; treat according to findings
  - If tissue diagnosis not possible, begin antifungal therapy with amphotericin B, liposomal amphotericin product, or voriconazole
  - Surgical excision indicated for locally destructive *Mucor* or *Aspergillus*
- **Diffuse infiltrate:**
  - Begin broad-spectrum antibiotics, plus trimethoprim-sulfamethoxazole (for *P. carinii*) and macrolide (for atypical bacterial pneumonia)
  - Reassess after 3 or 4 days:
    - Improved: Continue antibiotics for 2 weeks
    - Not improved: Obtain tissue (BAL or biopsy) and treat accordingly

■ Complications

- Empyema; pulmonary compromise including restrictive lung disease

Gastrointestinal Infections

■ Epidemiology

- Pathogens are acquired from endogenous flora, other persons, or contaminated food or water
- GI infections make up 5% to 7% of infections in those with fever/neutropenia

■ TABLE 20-2 Common Organisms Causing GI Tract Infection	
Symptom	**Potential Organisms**
Diarrhea	*Aeromonas* spp., *Campylobacter, C. difficile, E. coli, Listeria, Shigella, Salmonella, V. cholerae, Y. enterocolitica,* rotavirus, adenovirus, astroviruses, *Cryptosporidium, Cyclospora, Entamoeba, G. lamblia*
Esophagitis	*Candida* spp., HSV, CMV, other viruses, and many bacteria
Typhlitis	Anaerobes, enteric gram-negative bacteria, *C. difficile*
Peritonitis	Anaerobes, enteric gram-negative bacteria, *Clostridium* spp.
Hepatitis	Hepatitis viruses A, B, C, D, E, G; HSV, CMV, EBV, VZV
Hepatic abscess	Enteric gram-negative bacteria, *S. aureus, Candida* spp., *Mucor*
Perianal cellulitis	Enteric gram-negative bacteria, anaerobes, *Streptococcus* spp.

■ **Risk Factors**

- Disruption of gut mucosa (e.g., chemotherapy-induced mucositis)
- Alteration of normal gut microbial milieu: Antibiotics, surgery, mucositis
- Gut manipulation (e.g., rectal manipulation associated with perirectal abscess)

■ **Etiology (Table 20-2)/Pathogenesis**

- Changes in intestinal bacterial flora due to antibiotics, chemotherapy and other infections allow colonization by pathogenic organisms
- Disruptions in intestinal mucosa allow entry of potentially pathogenic organisms
- Immunosuppression allows pathogenic organisms to disseminate

■ **History**

- Abdominal pain, distension, diarrhea, constipation, blood in stool, fever
- Pain on swallowing, chest pain, reflux accompany esophagitis
- Jaundice, right upper quadrant pain suggest hepatic pathology
- Perianal pain, pain with defecating suggest perirectal lesion

■ **Physical Examination**

- Mouth: Erythema, ulcers, mucositis, thrush
- Abdomen: Distention, tenderness, masses, rebound, guarding, change in bowel sounds, perianal tenderness or fluctuant area
- Jaundice, hepatomegaly

■ **Additional Studies**

- Blood culture, CBCs, liver function tests
- Cultures of stool; antigen testing for viral pathogens, C. *difficile* toxin testing
- Abdominal imaging: Radiographs (look for obstruction, free air), CT scans (detect abscesses, areas of bowel well thickening)
- If diagnosis unclear, consider diagnostic endoscopy, colonoscopy, or liver biopsy

■ **Differential Diagnosis**

- Diarrhea caused by medications, radiation colitis, diet
- Esophagitis secondary to chemotherapy, acid reflux

■ **Management**

- Supportive care with fluids, intravenous nutrition if necessary
- Antimicrobials:
  - Bacterial infections: appropriate antibiotics
  - C. *difficile* diarrhea/colitis: Oral metronidazole (first line). Alternative: IV metronidazole or oral vancomycin
  - Herpetic stomatitis or esophagitis: Acyclovir intravenously
  - Candidal infections: Fluconazole or amphotericin B product
- Typhlitis (inflammation of the cecum): Conservative management with antimicrobials; surgery only for acute abdomen/ signs or perforation

■ **Complications**

- Chronic diarrhea; chronic hepatitis; esophagitis may lead to strictures

Human Immunodeficiency Virus Infection

Richard M. Rutstein, MD

HIV

- Epidemic continues despite recent decreases in mother-child transmission (MCT) and mortality/morbidity in areas with access to antiretroviral therapy (ART)
- Worldwide, approximately 1500 children infected daily. Most (more than 90%) have limited ART access

■ Epidemiology

- HIV transmitted via exposure to infected fluids: Blood (sharing contaminated needles, transfusion of tainted blood, rarely occupational exposure); body fluids (through anal or vaginal intercourse, breast-feeding)
- More than 95% of new pediatric cases occur secondary to MCT
- MCT may occur in utero, intrapartum, or postpartum (via breast-feeding)
- In the absence of breast-feeding, 80% of MCT occurs intrapartum

■ Rick Factors

- For MCT: High maternal viral load, low CD4 count, preterm delivery, chorioamnionitis, breast-feeding, prolonged rupture of membranes, vaginal delivery
- For non-MCT: Unprotected intercourse (receptive anal intercourse greater risk than receptive vaginal intercourse), exposure to infected blood

■ Etiology

- HIV-1 (99% of cases) and HIV-2, related retrovirus

■ Pathogenesis

- Prolonged period of clinical latency following infection (up to 10 years in adults)
- Active viral replication slowly overwhelms the immune system causing severe immunodeficiency. Frequent bacterial and opportunistic infections (OI) result

- The CD4 cell is the key target cell. Though all arms of the immune system are affected, the degree of immune dysfunction can be staged by measurement of the T-cell subset of CD4 percentage and number

■ History

- Inquire about risk factors in the parents (substance abuse, transfusions, STDs)
- Inquire about risk factors in the patient (sexual activity/abuse, substance abuse)
- Inquire about HIV testing in the parents
- Frequent invasive infections: pneumonia, arthritis, bacteremia
- Chronic or recurrent thrush
- Unexplained hepatitis, chronic diarrhea, poor growth

■ Physical Examination

- Poor growth statistics
- Generalized adenopathy, usually less than 2 cm
- Mild to moderate hepatosplenomegaly
- Chronic lung disease or hypoxemia at rest
- Acquired gross motor abnormalities or loss of developmental milestones

■ Diagnostic Evaluation

Who Should Be Tested?

- All pregnant women
- All sexually active adolescents should have routine HIV counseling and testing
- All children with parental history of: Sexually transmitted disease (STD); substance abuse, including non-IV cocaine use; bisexuality
- All infants or children with: Failure to thrive; generalized adenopathy; recurrent invasive bacterial disease; chronic parotitis; chronic diarrhea; unexplained hepatitis
- Children with atypical idiopathic thrombocytopenic purpura
- Loss of developmental milestones, if no other cause easily noted
- Chronic or recurrent thrush, especially after the age of 2 years

What Test to Use?

ANTIBODY TESTING

- HIV enzyme-linked immunosorbent assay (ELISA)
  - Sensitive and specific, though rarely false positives do occur
  - First screening test to confirm exposure in patient younger than 2 years

- IgG-based antibody, so all infants born to HIV-positive mothers will be ELISA positive at birth, by virtue of transplacental transfer of anti-HIV antibodies. Maternal antibodies detectable until 15 to 18 months of age
- HIV Western blot
  - Used as confirmatory test if ELISA positive. IgG based, more specific than ELISA
  - For patients older than 2 years, two positive ELISA and Western blot (WB) tests confirm HIV infection

VIRAL SPECIFIC TESTS
- HIV PCR DNA assay
  - High sensitivity (greater than 98%) and specificity when performed after 1 month of age
  - Because of 2% false-positive and false-negative rate, one positive does not prove HIV infection, and one negative does not rule out infection
- HIV blood culture
  - Also more than 98% sensitive and specific after 1 month of age but technically demanding, less available
- HIV PCR RNA quantitative assay (viral load, VL)
  - May be as sensitive as DNA assay, but more false positives at low values
  - If used for diagnosis, should be confirmed by DNA assay or blood coculture

Evaluation of Exposed Infants
- Perform, at a minimum, HIV PCR DNA assay or blood coculture at 1 month and 4 to 6 months of age. A positive test should be repeated immediately. Two positive viral specific test results confirms HIV infection
- If negative at 1 month and 4 to 6 months, patient is considered uninfected. Most consultants would still follow the infant until seroreversion (negative HIV antibody test), at 15 to 18 months of age
- For children and adolescents, two positive ELISA and WB tests confirms HIV infection

■ Additional Studies
- T-cell subsets
  - Measurement of CD4+ % and absolute cell number allows for staging of immunodeficiency. Use age-adjusted norms, as counts are high in infancy (normal 2500 to 3000/mm^3 in first year of life) and slowly fall to adult values (700 to 1000/mm^3) by age 7. In infected children, should be measured every 1 to 3 months

- Quantitative viral PCR (viral load, VL)
  - Measures viral RNA per milliliter. Range of tests from fewer than 40 copies per milliliter to more than 10 million per milliliter
  - In the first year of life, VLs are in 100,000 to 300,000 range prior to treatment. In older children, 50,000 to 100,000 range (as in most adults at time of diagnosis)
  - In general, the higher the VL, the greater the risk of progression to AIDS/death. Measure every 1 to 3 months initially but once stable on treatment, follow every 3 months

■ Differential Diagnosis

- Adenopathy/hepatosplenomegaly: Primary CMV, EBV, toxoplasmosis, lymphoma
- Frequent infections: Primary immune deficiency (see Chapter 22)

■ Management

- HIV-exposed infants
  - ZDV for first 6 weeks of life, then start TMP-SMX bid, 3 days/week
  - Test by PCR DNA assay at least at birth, 1 month, and 4 to 6 months
  - Continue TMP/SMX until 4-month PCR DNA assay is negative
  - Routine immunization schedule
- HIV-infected infants/children
  - Measure CD4 and viral load at least every 3 months
  - TMP/SMX in first year of life, and then based on CD4 counts
  - Initiate combination antiretroviral therapy for 1) all identified infected infants younger than 12 months; 2) CD4 count moderately suppressed for age; 3) HIV-related symptoms

Antiretroviral Agents

- Presently, there are five classes of antiretroviral agents, with a total of 19 FDA-approved antiretroviral drugs (Box 21-1)
- When initiating therapy, use combinations of three or four agents, from at least two classes
- Some drugs are coformulated to improve adherence (e.g., Combivir = ZDV + 3TC). Choices for children unable to swallow capsules/tablets are limited; many agents do not come in liquid form, some that do are unpalatable, or have high alcohol content
- Only 40% of children achieve viral loads of less than 40 copies per milliliter for more than 12 months

■ **BOX 21-1 Antiretroviral agents**

Nucleoside RTI
Zidovudine (ZDV, AZT)[a]
Lamivudine (3TC)[a]
Stavudine (d4T)[a]
Didanosine (ddI)[a]
Zalcitabine (ddC)
Tenofovir
Abacavir[a]
FTC

Nonnucleoside RTI
Nevirapine[a]
Delavirdine
Efavirenz[a]

Protease Inhibitors
Ritonavir[a]
Indinavir
Saquinavir
Nelfinavir
Lopinavir/ritonavir[a]
Amprenavir[a]
Atazanavir

Fusion Inhibitors
Enfuvirtide (T-20)

Nucleotide RTI
Tenofovir

As of May 1, 2004.
[a] Child-friendly formulation available as liquid, powder, or capsules that may be opened onto food.

- Each agent has unique short-term side effect profile. Long-term effects unknown
- All HIV-infected children require care of HIV treatment specialist to manage ART

■ **Complications**

- Recurrent invasive bacterial infections (especially with *Pneumococcus*)
  - Occur in up to 25% of HIV-infected patients
  - Due to severe B-cell dysfunction. May occur at any CD4 cell count level
  - Recurrent invasive bacterial infections are an indication to consider monthly IV gamma globulin

- *Pneumocystis carinii* pneumonia
  - Still most common severe complication of HIV in first year of life
  - Occurs in up to 20% of patients (peak incidence at 3 to 9 months)
  - After infancy, risk related to CD4% and counts. Require prophylaxis if CD4% is less than 15% to 20%, absolute CD4 less than 500 cells/mm^3 (younger than 5 years) or less than 200 cells/mm^3 (older than 5 years)
  - Think *P. carinii* in infant younger than 1 year, with tachypnea, hypoxemia, quiet rales (or no adventitial findings), CXR with interstitial/alveolar infiltrate. Elevated serum LDH reflects lung injury
  - Diagnosis: Identification of organism on histologic smears of lung fluid (obtained by BAL or aspiration), gives positive silver stain
  - Treatment is with high-dose IV TMP-SMX with or without adjunctive steroids for 3 weeks
  - Mortality close to 50% for first episode in infancy
  - Prophylaxis: TMP-SMX, 150 mg/m^2/d, 3 days/week. For patients allergic to TMP/SMX, use aerosolized pentamidine, or oral dapsone or atavoquone
- Progressive encephalopathy (PE)
  - Occurred in up to 25% of patients prior to advent of three- or four-drug combination therapy
  - Onset 9 to 18 months of age, rare after age 3 years
  - Key hallmark of disease is loss of previously acquired skills
  - May be rapid downhill progression, with death within 6 to 12 months of diagnosis. Some patients have a plateau phase without further developmental regression
  - Neuroimaging: Cerebral atrophy and basal ganglion calcifications
  - Seizures are infrequent in PE
- Lymphocytic interstitial pneumonitis (LIP)
  - Unique to perinatally acquired HIV. Onset around age 2 years
  - Chronic lung infiltration, most likely due to chronic activation from EBV infection
  - Several patterns: 1) Asymptomatic, noted on routine CXR as diffuse reticulonodular pattern; 2) slowly progressive chronic lung disease with hypoxemia, with or without wheezing; 3) slowly progressive pulmonary scarring, fibrosis
  - Lung biopsy confirms diagnosis
  - Treatment: For patients with symptomatic disease, long-term steroid therapy
- CMV end-organ disease

- Reported in 10% of patients, not as common as in adult HIV infection
- GI disease more common than retinitis; pulmonary disease uncommon
- *Candida* esophagitis
  - Usually seen in late-stage disease, those with CD4 counts less than $100/mm^3$
  - Presents with fever, dysphagia, chest pain, and, in most cases, oral thrush
  - Upper GI reveals suggestive pattern; endoscopy and biopsy for definitive diagnosis
- Disseminated *Mycobacterium avium*
  - Occurs late in disease; generally older than 5 years, with CD4 less than 100 cell/mm^3
  - Ultimately diagnosed in 5% to 10% of HIV-infected children
  - Presents with weeks of high fevers, weight loss, abdominal pain, diarrhea
  - Abdominal imaging frequently reveals prominent and diffuse lymphadenopathy
  - Diagnosis is by positive culture of normally sterile site (blood, node, bone marrow)
  - May take 3 to 4 weeks to grow in culture
- HIV-related lymphoma (less common than in adults; occurs in less than 2% of children)

■ Postexposure Prophylaxis

- Risk of transmission of HIV based on mechanism of exposure (Table 21-1)
- Postexposure prophylaxis (PEP) for occupational exposure based on retrospective studies; suggests 80% decrease in transmission rate if PEP given
- For high-risk occupational exposure from known HIV-positive patient, offer PEP
  - If high risk, start combination therapy for 4 weeks. Generally use three drugs, most frequently ZDV + 3TC (available as one tablet, to be taken twice per day) plus nelfinavir (5 tablets, twice per day). Drug regimen adjusted for index patients ART treatment history, resistance, viral load, as well as profile of exposed patient (pregnant, other medical issues)
  - For low/medium risk, consider two-drug therapy (fewer side effects) or no therapy
- Exposure to saliva, discarded needle on street, body fluid contact with intact skin, all considered *low risk*, generally no PEP indicated
- For sexual contact, consider exposure and risk of treatment. PEP for ongoing sexual relationship *not* appropriate except in

■ **TABLE 21-1** Risk of Transmission of HIV Based on Mechanism of Exposure

Risk (%)	Exposure
20–30	Mother to infant, if no therapy, no breast-feeding
10–15	Breast-feeding
0.5–3.2	Receptive anal intercourse
0.05–0.15	Receptive vaginal intercourse
0.3	Occupational exposure; needlestick from known HIV-positive patient
0.03–0.09	Insertive vaginal intercourse

instances of failure of barrier contraceptive method. For one-time sexual contact or sexual abuse, consider mechanism of exposure (anal, vaginal), trauma, and profile of perpetrator
- PEP unlikely to have benefit if initiated more than 72 hours after exposure
- Studies: 1) Baseline HIV ELISA/WB, CBC, liver function tests prior to starting PEP; 2) treat for 1 month (if indicated) with repeat HIV WLISA/WB at 6, 12, and 24 weeks after exposure (do not use HIV PCR DNA or RNA testing—too many false positives)
- Consultation HIV treatment specialist for individualized approach

22 Inherited Immune Deficiencies

Timothy Andrews, MD and Elena Elizabeth Perez, MD, PhD

Evaluation of Suspected Primary Immunodeficiency

- Inherited diseases of immune system function (single-gene defect or polygenic); more than 70 primary diseases known

■ Epidemiology

- Occur from approximately 1 in 10,000 to 1 in 2000 live births
- Affects humoral (B cell/antibody), cellular (T cell), or innate (phagocyte, complement) immunity alone or in combination

■ Risk Factors/Etiology (Box 22-1)

- Reasons to have a higher suspicion for an immune deficiency
  - Failure to thrive or severe nonatopic eczema
  - Chronic/recurrent infections: Otitis, sinusitis, pneumonia, severe diaper rash/thrush
  - Unusually severe infection or infection with low-virulence or opportunistic organism
  - Deep infections at multiple sites (e.g., liver abscess)
  - Family history of immunodeficiency, recurrent infections, consanguinity
  - Presence of autoimmune disease
  - Slow therapeutic response to infections despite appropriate therapy

■ History (Table 22-1)

- Date, duration, and site of infections
- How the diagnosis was established (e.g., cultures, radiologic imaging)
- Severity of the episode (e.g., shock, mechanical ventilation) and specific treatments
- Temporal relationships of previous episodes
- Birth history (separation of umbilical stump, requirement for blood product transfusion)
- Certain organisms should prompt consideration of a primary immune deficiency (see Box 22-1 for conditions)

■ **BOX 22-1 Categories of Primary Immune Deficiencies**

Humoral Deficiency (B cell)
Transient hypogammaglobulinemia of infancy[a]
X-linked agammaglobulinemia[a]
Common variable immunodeficiency[a]
IgA deficiency[a]
IgG subclass deficiency
Hyper-IgM (recessive form)

Cellular Immune Deficiency (T cell)
Interferon-γ IL-12 axis
Autoimmune polyglandular syndrome type 1

Combined Immune Deficiency (T cell and B cell)
Severe combined immunodeficiency[a]
22q11.2 deletion syndrome (velocardiofacial/DiGeorge)[a]
X-linked hyper-IgM syndrome
Autoimmune polyglandular syndrome type 1[a]
Wiskott-Aldrich syndrome[a]
Ataxia-telangiectasia
Defective natural killer cell function
X-Linked lymphoproliferative syndrome
Defective expression of major histocompatibility factor

Phagocyte Defect
Chédiak-Higashi syndrome[a]
Chronic granulomatous disease[a]
Cyclic neutropenia[a]
Hyper-IgE
Kostmann syndrome[a]
Leukocyte adhesion deficiency (type 1 or 2)[a]
Myeloperoxidase deficiency[a]
Specific granule deficiency[a]

Complement Deficiency
Early (C1–C4) component deficiencies
Terminal (C5–C9) component deficiencies
Properdin deficiency

[a] Discussed further in text or tables.

- *Staphylococcus aureus*: Humoral or combined deficiency, phagocyte defect
- *Streptococcus pneumoniae*: Combined or complement deficiency, asplenia, hemoglobinopathy
- *Neisseria* spp.: Humoral or complement deficiency
- *Aspergillus* spp.: Cellular or combined deficiency, or phagocyte defect

■ TABLE 22-1 Chief Complaints and Suspected Immune Deficiencies

Chief Complaint	Consider These Primary Immune Deficiencies
Chronic diarrhea	IgA deficiency, SCID, XLA
Recurrent otitis media/sinusitis	IgA deficiency, XLA, CVID
Recurrent pneumonia	IgA deficiency, XLA, CVID, hyper-IgE, CGD, SCID
Recurrent meningitis	Complement deficiency
Recurrent skin/soft-tissue infections	CGD
Fungal infections	T-cell/combined deficiency, CGD

- *Candida* spp.: Cellular or combined deficiency, or phagocyte defect
- *Mycobacterium avium*: Cellular or combined deficiency, phagocyte defect, HIV
- *Pneumocystis carinii*: Combined deficiency, phagocyte defect, HIV
- Enteroviruses (recurrent or severe): Humoral or combined deficiency

■ Physical Examination

- Search for previously unrecognized but significant physiologic or anatomic abnormalities. Examples:
  - Dysmorphic facial features (DiGeorge syndrome, hyper-IgE syndrome)
  - Gingivitis, ulcerations, periodontal disease (neutropenia)
  - Paucity of tonsillar tissue (X-linked agammaglobulinemia)
  - Petechiae (Wiskott-Aldrich) or seborrhea-like dermatitis (chronic granulomatous disease, Langerhans histiocytosis)

■ Diagnostic Evaluation

- **Basic screening for immunodeficiency:**
  - CBC with differential, noting absolute lymphocyte and neutrophil counts and peripheral blood smear
  - Quantitative immunoglobulins including IgG, IgA, IgM, and IgE
  - Titers to previous vaccines including tetanus, *Haemophilus influenzae* type B, diphtheria, and pneumococcus
  - Consider CH_{50}, nitroblue tetrazolium (NBT; see below), and HIV antibody
- **Tests for humoral immunodeficiency:** Quantitative immunoglobulins (IgG, IgA, IgM, IgE); antibody titers to vaccines; IgG subclasses (controversial)

- **Tests for cellular immunodeficiency**: Lymphocyte count; T-lymphocyte enumeration (flow cytometry); delayed-type hypersensitivity skin tests (limited value in infants younger than 1 year); thymic shadow on CXR; HIV antibody; mitogen/antigen lymphocyte stimulation
- **Tests for phagocyte defect**: Neutrophil count; NBT test or dichlorofluorescin if available; neutrophil chemotaxis assay
- **Tests for complement deficiency**: CH_{50}, AH_{50}; C3, C4, and other complement components when indicated

■ Differential Diagnosis

- **Consider diseases that may mimic or be associated with immunodeficiency**: Asthma, allergies, cystic fibrosis, inflammatory bowel disease, leukemia/lymphoma, protein-losing enteropathy, metabolic disorders
- **Consider causes of secondary immunodeficiency**: HIV/AIDS, malnutrition, chemotherapy, and steroid use

Humoral (Antibody) Deficiency

- Most common group of primary immune deficiencies
- Symptoms appear at 3 to 6 months of life as maternal antibodies wane below protective levels

Transient Hypogammaglobinemia of Infancy
- Abnormal delay in onset of antibody production
- Normal physiologic nadir is lower and more prolonged
- Affected patient may suffer recurrent upper respiratory tract infections
- Diagnosis: Serum IgG and IgA low with normal IgM
- Antibody response to protein antigens normal and circulating B cells normal
- Spontaneous resolution, usually by 2 to 3 years of age

X-linked Agammaglobulinemia (Bruton Agammaglobulinemia)
- Arrest of B-cell development at the pre–B-cell stage
- Mutation in Bruton's tyrosine kinase gene located on Xp22
- Occurs in 1 in 50,000 to 1 in 100,000
- Most common infections: Sinopulmonary infections (60% of affected children); gastroenteritis (35%); pyoderma (25%); arthritis (20%); meningitis (16%); sepsis (10%)
- Occasionally present with enteroviral encephalitis, viral hepatitis, or disseminated polio (live virus vaccine strain)
- Small to no lymphoid tissue (absent tonsils), arthritis, dermatomyositis-like syndrome
- Total absence or marked deficiency of all types antibody, including protective antibody

- Diagnosis: Absent or low (less than 2%) circulating B cells or lymphocytes with surface immunoglobulin
- Treat with monthly intravenous immune globulin (IVIG) to maintain normal serum IgG concentrations

Common Variable Immune Deficiency (CVID)
- Heterogeneous group of disorders with B-cell and T-cell dysfunction
- "Variable" reflects the wide age range at diagnosis and the degree of hypogammaglobinemia
- Recurrent otitis media, sinusitis, pneumonia, and bronchiectasis
- 50% with GI involvement chronic diarrhea, atrophic gastritis, pernicious anemia, nodular lymphoid hyperplasia
- Lymphoid hypertrophy including spleen and liver with secondary thrombocytopenia
- 25% with autoimmune disorders rheumatoid arthritis, hemolytic anemia, immune thrombocytopenia purpura, Guillain-Barré syndrome, autoimmune thyroid disease
- Diagnosis: Low immunoglobulin (Ig) levels, absent specific antibodies, variable T-cell function
- Treat with monthly IVIG. Prophylactic antibiotics benefit some patients with recurrent respiratory infections

IgA Deficiency
- Most common antibody deficiency with prevalence ranging from 1 in 400 (whites) to 1 in 5000 (Asians)
- In many with isolated IgA deficiency disease is asymptomatic; others develop recurrent sinopulmonary infections
- Associated with atopy and autoimmune disorders
- Diagnosis: Serum IgA concentration less than 7 mg/dL
- Risk for developing anti-IgA antibodies from blood products and subsequent anaphylaxis

Cellular and Combined Immune Deficiency

Severe Combined Immunodeficiency (SCID)
- Category of diseases resulting in abnormal lymphocyte number and function
- May be X-linked or autosomal recessive. Occurs in approximately 1 in 100,000 live births
- Manifestations include failure to thrive, recurrent/chronic respiratory infection, opportunistic or fungal infection
- Graft versus host disease rash from maternal T cells in some cases
- Initial management: Strict isolation, IVIG, no live vaccines, only irradiated CMV-negative blood products if necessary, trimethoprim-sulfamethoxazole (TMP-SMX) prophylaxis, search for bone marrow or stem cell donor

- Absolute lymphocyte count (ALC) is a big clue to the diagnosis. (ALC in newborns should be greater than 2000 to 11,000, and in 6- to 7-month olds greater than 4000.)
- Several genotypes/phenotypes. T cells may be low or absent. B cells may be normal, low, or absent

DiGeorge Syndrome (22q11.2 Deletion Syndrome, Velocardiofacial Syndrome)

- Wide variation in clinical disease; occurs in 1 in 2000 to 1 in 5000 live births
- Associated with defect in embryologic development of third and fourth pharyngeal pouches
- Thymus absent or hypoplastic (SCID-like or mild lymphopenia)
- Cardiac defects (conotruncal defects, atrial septal defect, ventricular septal defect, interrupted aortic arch, right-sided aortic arch)
- Possible associated defects: Esophageal atresia, bifid uvula, hypertelorism, low-set ears, palatal insufficiency
- Hypoparathyroidism, hypocalcemia
- Diagnosis: Fluorescent in situ hybridization (FISH) to detect 22q11.2 deletion
- Multidisciplinary approach to care: Speech pathology, genetics, cardiology, immunology, development
- No specific treatment unless profound defect necessitates thymic explants

Wiskott-Aldrich Syndrome

- Triad of immunodeficiency, eczema, and thrombocytopenia (platelets also small and defective)
- X-linked recessive inheritance; defect in *WASP* gene (product important for actin polymerization)
- Increased susceptibility to infection (*S. pneumoniae*, *P. carinii*, herpes virus)
- Poor antibody responses to polysaccharides
- Usual presentation in infancy with prolonged bleeding (circumcision, diarrhea, or bruising)
- Diagnosis: Specialized genetic testing to confirm diagnosis
- Human leukocyte antigen–identical sibling bone marrow transplants may be indicated

Phagocyte Disorders

Neutrophil Disorders (Table 22-2)

- Diminished neutrophil number or function (chemotaxis, phagocytosis, oxidative burst)

- Manifest as recurrent or severe infections with common bacteria and opportunistic pathogens (see "History" in section "Evaluation of Suspected Primary Immune Deficiency")
- Production disorders
  - **CBC with manual differential** to evaluate for decreased production (cyclic neutropenia, Kostmann syndrome, and Shwachman syndrome) and abnormal morphology (Chédiak-Higashi, specific granule deficiency)
  - Antineutrophil antibodies used to evaluate autoantibody neutropenia
- Functional disorders
  - **NBT and dihydroxyrhodamine 123 (DHR).** Both tests evaluate neutrophil oxidative burst. DHR with flow cytometry is more quantitative and requires less blood for evaluation

■ TABLE 22-2 Manifestation and Inheritance of Specific Neutrophil Disorders

Clinical Disease	Manifestations
Production Disorders	
Cyclic neutropenia	Recurrent fever, mucosal ulcers, cutaneous infections, lymphadenopathy, approximately 21-day cycle
Kostmann syndrome	Low neutrophil counts
Schwachman-Diamond syndrome	Metaphyseal dysostosis multiplex, pancreatic insufficiency, neutropenia
Function Disorders	
Chronic granulomatous disease	Recurrent infections catalase-positive bacteria, filamentous fungi, inflammatory complications, inflammatory bowel disease
Leukocyte adhesion deficiency type 1	Soft-tissue infection, tooth loss, omphalitis, delayed separation of umbilical cord, perirectal infections
Leukocyte adhesion deficiency type 2	Infections similar to type 1; in addition, short stature, mental retardation
Chédiak-Higashi syndrome	Recurrent infections cellulitis, abscess, otitis, periodontal disease with bone loss, oculocutaneous albinism, peripheral neuropathy, lymphoproliferative disorder
Myeloperoxidase deficiency	Most asymptomatic, rarely associated with severe candidiasis
Specific granule deficiency	Indolent skin and respiratory infections, otitis, and mastoiditis

- Neutrophil chemotaxis assay and neutrophil expression of **CD11b/18** evaluates disorders associated with decreased neutrophil chemotaxis and leukocyte adhesion defect
- **Bactericidal killing assay** evaluates neutrophil killing of *S. aureus* compared to normal control. *Detect any deficiency in neutrophil ability to recognize, phagocytose, and kill pathogens*

Macrophage Disorders

- Characterized by defects in intracellular killing. First infection usually before age 3 years
- Autosomal recessive inheritance; most common defect is in interferon-γ (IFN-γ) receptor 1 chain
- Increased susceptibility to intracellular infections, especially mycobacteria (*Mycobacterium avium* most common infection; others include *M. bovis*, *M. fortuitum*, and *M. tuberculosis*) and *Salmonella* species.
- 20% of patients with early death from infection
- Diagnosis usually requires testing to evaluate IFN-γ receptor expression and function
- Immunomodulator therapy: IFN-γ has shown benefit except in complete IFN-γ receptor defects

Infections in Other Immunocompromised Hosts

Marian G. Michaels, MD, MPH and Shruti M. Phadke, MD

Infections in Sickle Cell Disease

- Sickle cell disease (Hb SS): An autosomal recessive disorder
  - Valine is substituted for glutamine at the sixth position of the β-globin gene
  - Abnormal red blood cell structure and life span
- Increased risk for severe infections largely due to functional asplenia
- Other hemoglobinopathies are also at increased risk for infection but not to as large a degree as children with Hb SS
- Children with sickle trait (Hb AS) are at less risk for severe disease from *Plasmodium falciparum* in countries with endemic malaria

■ Epidemiology

- Highest risk for infection occurs during infancy through first 5 years of life
- Decreased risk during neonatal period due to persistent fetal hemoglobin
- Risk of invasive *Streptococcus pneumoniae* 100 to 500 times greater than normal child
  - Same serotypes of *S. pneumoniae* as those infecting healthy children
  - Increased risk of resistant *S. pneumoniae* because of frequent antibiotic use
  - Anticipate decreased frequency of *S. pneumoniae* with use of conjugate vaccine
- Conjugate vaccine against *Haemophilus influenzae* type b led to decreased disease
- Gram-negative rods (GNR) predominate in older children (e.g., *Salmonella*)
- Severe pneumonia or acute chest syndrome can occur with infection with *Mycoplasma pneumoniae* and *Chlamydia pneumoniae*

■ Risk Factors

- Splenic dysfunction: Lack of clearance of bacteria and decreased antibody synthesis

■ **TABLE 23-1 Etiology of Common Infections in Children with Sickle Cell Disease**

Syndrome	Common	Less Common
Bacteremia	*S. pneumoniae* *Salmonella* species Coagulase-negative staphylococci[a] *S. aureus*	*H. influenzae* *Candida* species[a] GNR á-Hemolytic streptococci *Neisseria meningitidis*
Osteomyelitis	*Salmonella* species *S. aureus* Enteric GNR	N/A
Pneumonia	*S. pneumoniae* *M. pneumoniae* *C. pneumoniae*	N/A
Other	Aplastic crisis: parvovirus B19	Urinary tract infections: enteric GNR

[a] Associated with central line presence.

- Defective alternate complement pathway: Decreased heat labile opsonic activity
- Local infarction and tissue necrosis
- Possible decrease in chemotaxis of neutrophils

■ **Etiology/Pathogenesis (Table 23-1)**

- Bacteremia with encapsulated organisms cannot be cleared efficiently
- Bone crisis leads to devitalized areas and increased risk of osteomyelitis
- Intravascular sickling of vessels of the bowel may lead to microischemia and damage the mucosal integrity leading to bacteremia from enteric organisms

■ **Physical Examination**

- Often deteriorate quickly
- Fever usually present
- Look for signs of specific infections. Most commonly: Sepsis, meningitis, pneumonia, osteomyelitis, urinary tract infection, and parvovirus B19 infection (see relevant chapters for specific examination findings)

■ **Additional Studies**

- CBC with differential and platelet count (severe anemia with low reticulocyte count in parvovirus B19; leukocytosis with other infections)
- Blood culture
- Urinalysis and urine culture
- Depending on physical examination and lab values, additional studies include:
  - Chest radiograph: 1) Respiratory symptoms present; 2) positive culture for *S. pneumoniae*
  - Radiographic studies to evaluate possible osteomyelitis: 1) Symptoms referable to joint or bone; 2) positive blood culture for *Salmonella* spp. or *S. aureus*
  - Lumbar puncture if CNS signs or symptoms

■ **Differential Diagnosis**

- Vaso-occlusive ischemia: Acute chest syndrome versus pneumonia; bone pain crisis versus osteomyelitis; stroke versus CNS infection; viral illness

■ **Management**

- Preventive strategies
  - Prophylaxis: Penicillin prophylaxis (daily) until at least 6 years of age
  - Vaccination against bacterial infections with routine childhood immunizations. Especially important: 1) *S. pneumoniae* (conjugate followed by polysaccharide after 2 years of age); 2) *H. influenzae* type B; 3) *Neisseria meningitidis*
- Aggressive evaluation of fevers for infectious cause
- Aggressive treatment of infections with antibiotics
- Bone marrow transplantation available for those with severe illness and frequent infections

Infections in Solid Organ Transplant Recipients

- Infections are a major cause of morbidity and mortality after transplantation
- The transplanted organ is often a major focus for the site of infection
  - Urinary tract infections or pyelonephritis after renal transplantation
  - Cholangitis and hepatitis after liver transplantation
  - Pneumonia after lung transplantation

- Some similarities exist regardless of the type of organ transplanted
  - Stereotypical timing of infections (see "Epidemiology")
  - Opportunistic infections

■ **Epidemiology/Risk Factors (Box 23-1)**

- Immunosuppression to prevent rejection
- Surgical manipulation
- Underlying disease
  - Cystic fibrosis patients infect new lungs with organisms from trachea/sinuses
  - Short-bowel syndrome, antibiotic-resistant organisms secondary to previous antibiotics
- Absence of primary immunity to many infectious agents prior to the time of transplantation (often age dependent)
- Donor-associated infections
  - Cytomegalovirus (CMV) (donor positive/recipient negative)

■ BOX 23-1 Typical Period of Time for Specific Infections Noted After Transplantation

Early (0–1 month)
Bacterial
  - Line infections
  - Surgical site
  - Urinary tract
  - Pneumonia
Candida spp.
Herpes simplex reactivation
Nosocomial infections

Middle (1–12 months)
Donor-associated/opportunistic
  - Cytomegalovirus
  - Epstein-Barr virus (PTLD)
  - *Pneumocystis* pneumonia
  - Nocardia
  - *Toxoplasma gondii*

Late (>12 months)
Community acquired
Bacterial (chronic rejection)
Aspergillus or other fungi
Epstein-Barr virus (PTLD)[a]

[a] EBV/PTLD ongoing risk in late period although less than in middle period.

- Epstein-Barr virus (EBV) (donor positive/recipient negative)
- *Toxoplasma gondii* (donor positive/recipient negative): Heart transplantation has highest risk
- Seasonal risks:
  - Winter months: Respiratory syncytial virus, influenza, parainfluenza (most severe early after transplantation)
  - Summer months: West Nile virus transmission from donor or blood products

■ Pathogenesis

- Opportunistic infections arise due to immunosuppression particularly affecting the T cells
- Donor-associated infections
  - Infectious agents in the donor are transmitted to the new host from the graft or accompanying blood cells or from transfusions
  - Infectious agents that can be maintained asymptomatically in the donor, especially 1) viruses (CMV, EBV, HIV, HBV, HCV); 2) parasites (*T. gondii*); 3) endemic fungi (histoplasmosis)
- Bacterial pathogens
  - Early after transplantation, most common: 1) Surgical wound sites; 2) invasive catheters (central venous, urethral, or tracheal intubation); 3) nosocomial transmission
  - Late after transplantation associated with chronic rejection
- Community-acquired viruses: Seasonal and may be nosocomial
  - Usually most severe if early after transplantation

■ History

- Time after transplantation
- Serologic status of recipient and donor
- Type of immunosuppression
- Type of antimicrobial prophylaxis

- Previous infections
- Type of transplant
- Presence of catheters
- Immunosuppression levels
- Exposures

■ Additional Studies

- Modifications based on type of transplant, history, infection suspected, and findings on physical examination
- Fever workup should include:
  - CBC with differential and platelet count
  - Blood culture
  - Viral cultures and relevant tests for likely viruses (see "Diagnostic Virology")

- Consideration of biopsy of graft
- Radiographs of chest and abdomen to identify masses or enlarged nodes
- Biopsy and cultures (bacterial, viral, fungal, mycobacterial) of nodes or masses
- Nucleic acid studies for patients at risk for EBV/CMV/ opportunistic infections

▪ Differential Diagnosis
- Rejection, drug reaction, malignancy

▪ Management
- Treatment aimed at specific infectious agent
- Decrease or discontinuation of immunosuppression
- Biopsy whenever possible to rule out rejection and determine specific infectious agent

Infections in Patients with Cystic Fibrosis

- Cystic fibrosis is an autosomal recessive disease
  - Most common life-shortening inherited disease among Caucasians
  - Found in all ethnic groups
  - Characterized by chronic and recurrent sinopulmonary infections and maldigestion resulting in poor weight gain and growth
- Chronic bacterial infection of lungs and sinuses
  - Significant contributor to progressive small airways obstruction and fibrosis and destruction of lung parenchyma

▪ Epidemiology
- Incidence: Northern European descent: 1 in 3200; African descent: 1 in 17,000; Asian descent: 1 in 90,000
- Genetics:
  - Gene (on long arm of chromosome 7) codes for a protein that functions in chloride conductance (Cystic Fibrosis Transmembrane Conductance Regulator, or CFTR)
  - More than 1000 gene mutations known but ΔF508 is present in 70% of affected patients

▪ Etiology
- Chronic infection/inflammation of the lower respiratory tract and sinuses
  - *S. aureus*, nontypeable *H. influenzae*, *Pseudomonas aeruginosa*

- Other gram-negative species (*Escherichia coli*, *Klebsiella pneumoniae*, *Stenotrophomonas maltophilia*, *Burkholderia cepacia*)
- *Aspergillus*: Allergic bronchopulmonary aspergillosis (ABPA)

■ **Pathogenesis**

- Abnormal CFTR structure/function leads to increased viscosity of secretions, particularly in the exocrine pancreas and lungs
- Mechanism of lung disease: 1) Inspissation of secretions; 2) bronchial obstruction; 3) chronic suppurative infection; 4) progressive airways inflammation; 5) bronchiectasis

■ **History**

- Community-acquired viral respiratory infections trigger pulmonary exacerbations
- Increasing fatigue, worsening exercise tolerance
- Worsening cough, increasing sputum production
- Signs and symptoms of worsened malabsorption (e.g., bulky, greasy, malodorous stools and weight loss)

■ **Physical Examination**

- General appearance, vital signs, and growth parameters
  - Respiratory rate and oxyhemoglobin saturation
  - Weight loss with pulmonary exacerbations and pneumonia
- Signs of respiratory distress and dyspnea
  - Nasal flaring and retractions (intercostal and abdominal)
  - Use of accessory muscles of respiration
- Contour and shape of thorax
  - Barrel chest in patients with chronic lung disease results from progressive smaller airways obstruction
- Palpation and percussion of hyperinflated lungs
- Auscultation (air entry; prolongation of expiratory phase; fine, end-inspiratory crackles)
- Other pertinent physical findings: 1) Nasal polyps are present in 10% to 15% of patients; 2) sinus tenderness with associated symptoms; 3) hepatosplenomegaly resulting from liver cirrhosis and portal hypertension; 4) digital clubbing

■ **Additional Studies**

- Sputum culture for bacterial pathogens with antibiotic susceptibilities
- Pulmonary function tests for changes in spirometric parameters
- Chest radiographs for evidence of bronchiectasis, peribronchial thickening and cuffing, hyperinflation, and infiltrates

■ Management

- Antibiotics to treat chronic airway infection and inflammation
  - Oral, inhaled, or intravenous routes
  - Antipseudomonal treatment requires a combination of active antibiotic groups (e.g., β-lactam and aminoglycoside)
- Mobilization of viscous, inspissate secretions: 1) Airway clearance techniques; 2) inhaled mucus-thinning agents
- Goals of therapy: Control chronic infection and prevent progression of lung disease

■ Complications

- Related to infection
  - Atelectasis from impacted mucous secretions
  - Hemoptysis can result from chronic inflammation and the development of tortuous collateral vessels of the bronchial arteries
  - Other allergic/inflammatory processes (e.g., ABPA)
- Related to frequent use of antibiotics (e.g., drug-resistant pathogens, renal and audiologic dysfunction resulting from frequent aminoglycoside use)
- Related to progressive airways obstruction (e.g., pneumothorax can result with rupture of blebs; respiratory failure and cor pulmonale in advanced stages of lung disease)

Biowarfare Agents

Andrew L. Garrett, MD and Fred M. Henretig, MD

- Regardless of your level of experience, you may be the first person to suspect an exposure to a biologic warfare (BW) agent. Your response to such a situation may determine whether the incident is controlled promptly or whether it evolves into a large-scale epidemiologic catastrophe.
- The most likely BW agents are discussed below.

Anthrax

- *Bacillus anthracis*: Gram-positive, encapsulated, aerobic, spore-forming rod
- Primarily a zoonotic pathogen in herbivores

■ Pathogenesis

- Three mechanisms of infection: 1) Inoculation of open skin; 2) inhalation; 3) ingestion
- Human to human transmission is possible in cutaneous form, otherwise unlikely

■ History/Physical Examination

- Incubation usually 1 to 7 days but may be up to 6 weeks for inhalational form

Cutaneous (Most Common)

- Papule → vesicular lesion → black scab (eschar) → (rarely) lethal systemic infection
- Lesions are painless and typically located on hands/arms at site of broken integument

Inhalational

- Gradual onset of fever, malaise, nonproductive cough, fatigue, and chest pain
- May have transient improvement over 2 to 3 days
- Subsequent sudden development of severe respiratory symptoms: Dyspnea, diaphoresis, cyanosis, stridor; 50% develop hemorrhagic meningitis

Gastrointestinal
- Initially fever, nausea, anorexia then abdominal pain, hematemesis, bloody diarrhea

Oropharyngeal
- Neck swelling from lymphadenopathy can compromise airway
- Throat pain, dysphagia, and ulcers at base of tongue

■ **Additional Studies**
- Routine culture of blood (inhalational, GI disease), CSF (meningitis), or lesion (cutaneous) may demonstrate *B. anthracis*
- Toxin detection assay in cases of bacteremia may be helpful
- CXR may show *widened mediastinum*, pleural effusion, or infiltrate
- Culture of nasal swabs used for epidemiologic data collection but not for diagnosis

■ **Differential Diagnosis**
- Cutaneous: Tularemia, bacterial skin infection, brown recluse spider bite
- Inhalational: Dissecting aortic aneurysm, superior vena cava syndrome
- GI: Acute abdomen, food poisoning

■ **Management**
- **Ciprofloxacin** *or* **doxycycline**; *plus* (for inhalational anthrax) **clindamycin** (may reduce toxin production). Treat for 2 months
- Weaponized forms may be engineered to be resistant to common antibiotics
- Begin treatment as soon as disease is suspected. Mortality: Inhalational almost always fatal; cutaneous, 20% fatal; GI, 50% fatal when untreated
- Prophylaxis for suspected aerosol exposures is with **ciprofloxacin** for 2 months. Alternative is **doxycycline**. Consider **amoxicillin** for documented sensitive strains
- Vaccination possible if high risk of exposure (e.g., military, animal workers)

Plague

- *Yersinia pestis*: Gram-negative, rod-shaped, non-sporulating bacterium
- Primarily a zoonotic pathogen in rodents; enzootic in southwestern United States

■ Pathogenesis

- *Primary* pneumonic plague (contagious) likely from aerosolized *Y. pestis*. Most likely form if used as a biowarfare agent.
- *Bubonic* plague (non-contagious) transmitted by infected fleas. May progress to *secondary* pneumonic or septicemic plague

■ History/Physical Examination

Pneumonic

- Incubation 1 to 3 days in primary pneumonic disease, longer in secondary
- Rapid onset of severe respiratory symptoms: High fever, chills, malaise, myalgias, headache progress over 24 hours to *bloody sputum* and cough

Bubonic

- Incubation typically 2 to 10 days
- Acute onset of high fever, malaise, myalgias, headache, nausea and vomiting
- Painful lymphadenopathy (bubo) develops concurrently in extremity bitten by flea
- Painful hepatosplenomegaly; skin lesions in lymphatic drainage area of bubo

Septicemic

- Secondary in 25% of those who develop bubonic plague
- Acral thromboses, necrosis, gangrene, and disseminated intravascular coagulation (DIC) as part of endotoxin release; 6% develop meningitis

■ Additional Studies

- CXR: Bilateral infiltrates in pneumonic plague
- Leukocytosis with more than 80% neutrophils. DIC may occur
- Identification of a coccobacillus in lymph node aspirate, sputum, blood, or CSF
- Organism grows slowly in routine culture medium, so enzyme-linked immunosorbent assay F1 *Y. pestis* antigen detection confirms the diagnosis

■ Differential Diagnosis

- Community-acquired pneumonia, hantavirus pulmonary syndrome, rickettsiosis, meningococcemia, pneumonic plague, ricin or staphylococcal enterotoxin B

■ Management

- **Gentamicin** or **streptomycin**. In meningitis, consider adding chloramphenicol

- Prophylaxis **doxycycline** for 7 days. Alternate: **ciprofloxacin, tetracycline,** or **chloramphenicol**
- Vaccination is not available in the United States

Tularemia

- *Francisella tularensis*: Gram-negative coccobacillus
- Primarily zoonotic disease. Known as "rabbit fever" or "deer fly fever" and associated with animal workers, trappers, and those exposed to insect vectors

■ Pathogenesis
- Biologic attack (aerosolized release) would lead to either primary pneumonic form (contagious) or typhoidal form with or without secondary pneumonic component

■ History/Physical Examination
- Incubation 3 to 5 days (ranges up to 3 weeks)
- **Pneumonic**: Severe atypical pneumonia with bloody pleural effusion
- **Typhoidal**: Acute onset of symptoms: High fever, malaise, myalgias, occasionally shock
  - On examination, hepatosplenomegaly but sparse lymphadenopathy
  - Pneumonia from hematogenous seeding develops in 30% to 80%

■ Additional Studies
- Elevated creatine phosphokinase (rhabdomyolysis) with typhoidal form
- CXR: Typical or interstitial pneumonia possibly with pleural effusion
- Polymerase chain reaction (PCR) useful from swabs of ulcers
- Bacteria may be cultured from blood, lesion swabs, and sputum, but require specific media and precautions given risk of spread of tularemia
- Antibodies present 11 to 21 days after onset of symptoms.

■ Differential Diagnosis
- Severe pulmonary infections: *Mycoplasma*, plague
- Typhoidal illnesses: Malaria, salmonella, rickettsia

■ Management
- **Streptomycin** or **gentamicin** for 7 to 14 days

- Prophylaxis with doxycycline for 2 weeks if exposed but infection is asymptomatic
- Vaccination via a live attenuated product is available for laboratory workers

Smallpox

- Caused by the Orthopoxvirus variola; two forms: *major* and *minor*
- Endemic disease eliminated in 1980 by World Health Organization, but integrity of the few remaining stockpiles of the virus is unknown

■ Pathogenesis

- Infection by inhalation of aerosolized virus or indirect contact (contaminated fomites)

■ History/Physical Examination

- Incubation period: 7 to 19 days
- Febrile prodrome: 1 to 4 days before rash; fever, headache, myalgias, backache, vomiting, or abdominal pain
- Evolution of lesions from macules to papules to pustules (each stage lasts 1 to 2 days)
- Classic lesions: Deep-seated, firm, round, well-circumscribed vesicles or pustules that may become umbilicated or confluent
- Centrifugal distribution: Lesions concentrate on face and distal extremities. On any one part of body, all lesions are in the same stage of development
- Patients infectious from rash onset until scab separation (7 to 10 days after rash onset)
- Milder illness in variola minor infections and in previously immunized individuals

■ Additional Studies

- Diagnosis by electron microscopy of vesicular scrapings. Consider silver staining or PCR of specimens. Specimens should be handled at one of a small number of federal laboratories

■ Differential Diagnosis

- Varicella, monkeypox, cowpox, erythema multiforme, contact dermatitis

■ Management

- Initial outbreak response focuses on containment of symptomatic patients

- In the event of a documented case, vaccination of the public via scarification may contain an outbreak. It may be useful up to several days after exposure
- Pre-event vaccination of certain groups (military, physicians, etc.) is controversial. Live vaccinia virus currently used, but tissue cell culture vaccines are in development. Potential vaccine-related complications include cardiac disease and death
- Vaccinia immune globulin may treat severe side effects of vaccination
- Antivirals (e.g., cidofovir) are being investigated for use in smallpox

Viral Hemorrhagic Fevers

- Viral hemorrhagic fever (VHF): Potential bioweapon due to aerosol infectivity
- Four families of virus and some of their respective illnesses:
  - *Arenavirus*: Machupo, Lassa, Argentine hemorrhagic fever
  - *Bunyavirus*: Hantavirus, Congo-Crimean fever, Rift Valley fever
  - *Filovirus*: Ebola, Marburg
  - *Flavivirus*: Yellow fever, dengue
- Oubreak of Ebola v Reston among primates imported to the United States in 1989 inspired the book *The Hot Zone*. This strain was not pathogenic in humans

■ Epidemiology/Pathogenesis

- *Arenavirus* (carried by rodents): Inhaled dust contaminated by rodent waste. Endemic in areas of Central America and West Africa
- *Bunyavirus* (carried by ticks, rodents, mosquitoes): Inhaled dust contaminated by rodent waste or by infected arthropod or insect bite. Endemic in Africa, Europe, Asia. Hantavirus, carried by rodents, is seen in the southwestern United States
- *Filovirus* (carrier unknown): Infectious body fluids and in some cases by respiratory route. Endemic in areas of Africa, but periodically emerges into humans and primates
- *Flavivirus* (carried by mosquitoes and ticks): Infectious by bite of infected carrier
- Common pathophysiology: Degradation of the vascular system and coagulopathy

■ History/Physical Examination

- Fever, myalgias, weakness
- Microvascular degradation, coagulopathy, and complement system activation

- Conjunctival injection, hypotension, flushing, petechial lesions, edema
- Some progress to shock, mucous membrane hemorrhage, DIC, multiorgan failure

■ Additional Studies

- Clusters of unusual diseases will likely be the first signs. Not all cases of VHF will be a bioweapon attack, as these diseases are endemic in some locations.
- *Thrombocytopenia, leukopenia,* elevated hepatic enzymes, proteinuria, and hematuria
- Enzyme-linked immunoassays may provide rapid diagnosis of the viremia in some cases. Viral culture may also diagnose a suspected VHF virus

■ Differential Diagnosis

- Parasitemia (e.g., malaria), typhoid fever, shigellosis, leptospirosis, rickettsiosis, gram-negative sepsis, leukemia, systemic lupus erythematosus, idiopathic thrombocytopenic purpura

■ Management

- Patients require negative pressure isolation. Management primarily supportive
- Outbreak control relies on containment of patients and their infectious byproducts
- Some patients with VHF virus infections may benefit from **ribavirin** use
- Argentine hemorrhagic fever patients may benefit from convalescent serum use
- Vaccination is limited to the yellow fever vaccine. See the Centers for Disease Control recommendations at *www.cdc.gov* for current guidelines for international travel

Botulinum

- A potent neurotoxin formed by *Clostridium botulinum*. Inhaled toxin produces symptoms identical to food-borne botulism

■ Pathogenesis

- Blocks neuromuscular transmission by preventing release of acetylcholine

■ History/Physical Examination

- Symptoms appear 12 to 36 hours after exposure

- Initial manifestations: Autonomic effects (mydriasis, ileus, constipation, dry mouth) and cranial nerve palsies (diplopia, ptosis)
- Later manifestations: Symmetric descending flaccid musculoskeletal paralysis and respiratory failure

■ Additional Studies

- Clinical diagnosis but may have transiently positive edrophonium (Tensilon) test
- Toxin neutralization assay in mice identifies botulinum toxin in serum and stool

■ Differential Diagnosis

- Guillain-Barré syndrome, tick paralysis, myasthenia gravis, nerve agent, cholinergic intoxication, and food-borne botulism

■ Management

- Respiratory support and dependent care for up to several months
- Botulinum antitoxin (BAT) is available and neutralizes circulating toxin but will not reverse symptoms. A vaccine is available but not to the general public. Prophylactic use of BAT is not recommended

25 Prevention of Infection

Jean O. Kim, MD

Active Immunization

- Stimulating humoral or cellular immunity by administering vaccine or toxoid
- Immunologic response by host similar to that induced by natural infection but with fewer complications
- Protection may be lifelong or short term
- Usually administered before exposure to infectious agent, but may be given following exposure (see "Chemoprophylaxis")

Types of Vaccines
- **Live attenuated:** Weakened infectious agents that cause trivial active infections (varicella, oral polio, and measles, mumps, rubella vaccines)
- **Inactivated:** Killed infectious agents that do *not* cause active infections
- **Subunit preparations:** Components (proteins or polysaccharides) of infectious agents
- **NOTE: Polysaccharide antigens produce suboptimal antibody response in hosts younger than 2 years; protein conjugation improves antibody production significantly**
- Recommended childhood and adolescent vaccine schedule available at the Centers for Disease Control and Prevention (CDC) website (*www.cdc.gov/mmwr*)

Adverse Events
- Related to causative component of vaccine: 1) Active antigen: infectious agent or part thereof; 2) preservatives: antibiotics or chemical stabilizers; 3) suspension fluid: products used in tissue cell culture (e.g., egg antigens or gelatin)
- The Vaccine Adverse Event Reporting System (VAERS) is a method for surveillance of clinical events occurring after immunization. Common adverse events following routine immunizations include:
  - Diphtheria-tetanus-pertussis (DTP): All side effects are much *less* common with DTaP now in use
    - Fever greater than 40.5°C within 48 hours after DTP (0.3%)

- Hypotonic-hyporesponsive episodes: varies from 3.5 to 291 episodes per 100,000 doses
- Prolonged crying for 3 hours or more after DTP vaccination: One episode per 100 doses
- Measles-mumps-rubella (MMR):
  - Fever 39.4°C or higher lasting 1 or 2 days in the 6 to 12 days following MMR vaccination in 5% to 15% of recipients
  - Transient thrombocytopenia in 1 per 25,000 to 40,000 MMR vaccine recipients
- Varicella:
  - Mild varicella-like illness (typically 15 to 30 vesicles) in 1% to 4%
  - Fever 38.0°C or higher in 10% of adolescent and adult varicella vaccine recipients
- More information about the VAERS system can be found on the web at www.vaers.org. A table of reportable/reported adverse vaccine reactions can be found at *http://www.vaers.org/reportable.htm*. In addition, reports can be phoned in to 1-800-822-7967.

Passive Immunization

- Administration of preformed protection (e.g., antibody) to an infectious agent to a host.
- Indicated in the following:
  - Pre-exposure: The patient is unable to mount an antibody response to an infectious agent due to congenital or acquired immunodeficiency
  - Postexposure: Exposure to an infectious agent placed patient at high risk for complication from disease
  - Disease: Both infectious and noninfectious diseases where antibody provides effective treatment

Products (Tables 25-1 and 25-2)
- Immune globulin (IG): Pooled plasma from adult donors; contains more than 95% IgG and trace amounts of IgA and IgM. Administer intravenously (IVIG) or intramuscularly with doses depending on indication (see *2000 Red Book*, published by the American Academy of Pediatrics).
- Adverse events related to IVIG occur in 5% of infusions
  - Common clinical reactions include the following: Fever, chills, headache, myalgia, nausea, vomiting, aseptic meningitis, acute renal failure, and vasomotor changes such as tachycardia and hypertension

■ **TABLE 25-1 Indications for Prophylaxis Using Immune Globulin Products**

Product[a]	Preventative Indication(s)
Intravenous immune globulin (IVIG)	Postexposure prophylaxis for hepatitis A and measles
Hepatitis B immune globulin (HBIG)	Hepatitis B virus exposed neonates or other susceptible hosts. Also administer active hepatitis B vaccine
Varicella-zoster immune globulin (VZIG) Administer IM. • May use IVIG if IM injections contraindicated	Varicella exposure in susceptible hosts: 1) Immunocompromised patients without history of VZV 2) Pregnant women without VZV antibodies 3) Newborn whose mother had VZV onset within 5 days before or 48 hours after delivery 4) Hospitalized premature infant 28 weeks or more gestation with negative maternal history of VZV *or* less than 28 weeks gestation or weight 1000 g or less, regardless or maternal history
Cytomegalovirus immune globulin (CMV IG)	CMV-seronegative kidney or liver transplant recipients of CMV-positive organs
Respiratory syncytial virus immune globulin (RSV IVIG) or RSV monoclonal antibody[b]	Prevention of RSV infection in children younger than 2 years requiring medical therapy for chronic lung disease or born 32 weeks or less gestation

[a] See "Infections Following Bites" (Chapter 16) for discussion of rabies immune globulin.
[b] RSV monoclonal antibody does not interfere with administration of live virus vaccines; administer IM.

■ **TABLE 25-2 Therapeutic Indications for Immune Globulin Products**

Product	Therapeutic Indication(s)
Intravenous immune globulin (IVIG)	Replacement for IgG deficiency; Kawasaki disease; hepatitis A exposure; immune-mediated thrombocytopenia; Guillain-Barré syndrome
Cytomegalovirus immune globulin (CMV IG)	CMV IG may be synergistic in managing CMV pneumonia in bone marrow transplant patients when given with ganciclovir
Botulinum immune globulin (HBIG; human botulinum antitoxin)	Infantile botulism; use equine-derived antitoxin in hypersensitivity-tested adults if HBIG not available
Tetanus immune globulin (TIG)	Treatment for tetanus: administer both intramuscularly and locally around wound. Use in conjunction with antibiotic (metronidazole or penicillin G) to reduce the number of vegetative forms of *Clostridium tetani*

- Alleviation of infusion-related side effects: Reduce rate or volume of infusion or pretreat with hydrocortisone 1 to 2 mg/kg 30 minutes prior to infusion with or without diphenhydramine
- Anaphylaxis may occur in persons with IgA deficiency due to reaction of anti-IgA antibodies to small amounts of IgA in some IVIG preparations
- In 1994 an outbreak of hepatitis C virus (HCV) occurred in recipients of one IVIG product. As IVIG is a human blood product, it is screened for HIV, HBV, and, now, HCV.

Chemoprophylaxis

• Administering antibiotics to prevent infection

Postexposure Prophylaxis
• Indicated to prevent infection by highly contagious and highly pathogenic organisms (Table 25-3)

TABLE 25-3 Postexposure Prophylaxis Regimens	
Disease[a]	Management of Exposure
Meningococcus infection	• Rifampin (2 days), ceftriaxone (1 dose), or ciprofloxacin (1 dose)
TB	• INH; add rifampin if exposed to INH-resistant TB individual • Place tuberculin skin test initially and repeat at 3 months; if positive, continue therapy for 9 months, if negative at 3 months discontinue therapy
Pertussis	• Erythromycin estolate (14 days). Azithromycin (5–7 days) may be as effective
Hepatitis B infection	• None if exposed person has positive HBsAb • HBIG once and begin HBV series if exposed person never vaccinated; HBIG twice if exposed person vaccinated but has negative titer • Evaluation: HBsAg, HBsAb, and liver enzymes at baseline, 3, and 6 months
Hepatitis C infection	• No prophylaxis available. Evaluation: HCV Ab, liver enzymes at baseline, 3, and 6 months
Influenza	• Amantadine, rimantadine, or oseltamivir for 5 days • Also give influenza vaccine if unvaccinated
Varicella[b]	• Varicella vaccine up to 5 days after exposure • VZIG may be given (see Table 25-1)

[a] See Chapter 21 for discussion of HIV postexposure prophylaxis.
[b] Susceptible, exposed health care workers should be furloughed from days 8 to 21 following exposure. VZIG recipients should be furloughed until day 28.

- Often intended to decrease colonization with pathogen, thus preventing infection
- May include a combination of antibiotics, antiretroviral agents, vaccine, and/or immunoglobulin

Infection Control

- Infection control programs are mandatory for all health care organizations
- Policies based on recommendations of national associations including the Centers for Disease Control and Prevention (CDC), the Society for Healthcare Epidemiology in America (SHEA),

■ TABLE 25-4 Disease Transmission and Precautions

Mode of Transmission		Isolation Precaution
Standard	Applicable to all body fluids, secretions, and excretions except sweat. Consider all patients as possibly infectious for blood-borne pathogens, such as HIV	• Hand hygiene (hand washing or use of alcohol-based product) between patients and after removal of other protective gear • Gloves to be worn when touching blood, body fluids, or contaminated items • Masks and/or eye protection if generation of spray or splash of fluids possible • Gowns (nonsterile) to prevent soiling of clothing and protect skin during procedures that create splash or spray
Contact	Direct (host-to-host) or indirect (with intermediary contaminated object) contact between infectious agent and host required for transmission	• Private room, if available; if not, cohort patients • Gloves and gowns • Hand hygiene following glove and gown removal
Droplet	Infection is spread by propulsion of larger droplets directly onto mucosal surfaces (conjunctivae, mouth, nose) over short distance	• Private room, if available; if not, cohort patients or place minimum 3 feet away from other patients • Masks within 3 feet of patient
Airborne	Infection may be spread by aerosolization of small (5 im or less) droplets remaining suspended in air for prolonged periods	• Private room in hospital. • Negative air pressure ventilation with 6–12 air changes per hour • Masks (for TB, N-95 fitted masks)

■ TABLE 25-5 Type of Precaution Based on Organism	
Precaution	**Clinical Examples**
Standard	All patient care
Contact	*Clostridium difficile* colitis; draining abscess; enteroviruses; hepatitis A, herpes simplex virus (mucocutaneous); herpes zoster,[a] lice (pediculosis); multidrug-resistant bacteria,[b] parainfluenza, respiratory syncytial virus, rotavirus; scabies; shigellosis; viral hemorrhagic fever
Droplet	Adenovirus; *Bordetella pertussis*; *Haemophilus influenzae* type b; influenza; mumps; *Mycoplasma pneumoniae*; *Neisseria meningitides*; parvovirus B19; rubella; streptococcal pharyngitis
Airborne	Measles; smallpox; tuberculosis; varicella-zoster virus

[a] Immunocompromised hosts with herpes zoster infection and immunocompetent hosts with disseminated disease may shed varicella virus from the respiratory tract and require contact plus airborne isolation for the duration of illness.
[b] Methicillin-resistant *Staphylococcus aureus*, vancomycin-resistant enterococci, glycopeptide intermediate/resistant *S. aureus*, extended-spectrum β-lactamase–producing gram-negative bacteria.

and the Joint Commission on Accreditation of Healthcare Organizations (JCAHO).

- Traditionally infection control programs focused on nosocomial infections. However, basic principles now applied to settings outside of the hospital, including outpatient clinics, long-term care facilities, and home health

General Principles of Isolation

- **Goal** is to limit transmission from infected host to other persons
- **Mode** of transmission and transmissibility from host to host determine type of isolation
- **Clinical presentation** may also influence type of precautions taken
- **Duration** of isolation determined by duration and degree of shedding from infected host
- Consult hospital infection control department for specific recommendations (Tables 25-4 and 25-5)

Other Components of Infection Control

- **Surveillance:** Infection control departments track infection rates and trends and attempt to reduce rates of specific infections. Examples: Nosocomial pneumonia, methicillin-resistant *Staphylococcus aureus* infections, surgical site infections
- **Reporting specific communicable diseases to public health authorities:** Certain infections are a public health concern and should be investigated beyond the hospital setting. Identification of these diseases may be the first indication of local outbreaks. Examples include tuberculosis, pertusis, and measles

A

Opportunities in Pediatrics and Pediatric Infectious Diseases

Pediatric Residency Training

There are currently 213 accredited categorical pediatric residency training programs in the United States and 16 accredited programs in Canada. Each year 2500 to 3000 residents begin pediatric training. At the completion of a 3-year residency, candidates may take the General Pediatrics Certifying Examination to become a board-certified pediatrician.

Pediatric Subspecialty Training

Each year 25% to 30% of graduating pediatric residents begin subspecialty fellowship training. Possible pediatric fellowship choices include the following:

- Adolescent medicine
- Behavioral/developmental pediatrics
- Cardiology
- Critical care
- Emergency medicine
- Endocrinology
- Gastroenterology
- Hematology-oncology
- Infectious diseases
- Neonatal-perinatal medicine
- Nephrology
- Pharmacology-toxicology
- Pulmonology
- Rheumatology
- Sports medicine

The duration of additional training in the standard fellowship pathway is 3 years. This is generally divided into 1 year of clinical training followed by 2 years of scholarly activity. These activities include either clinical or laboratory research. Some fellows augment their clinical research training with a master's degree in public health, biostatistics, or clinical epidemiology. An alternative pathway includes 2 years of general pediatric residency training ("fast tracking"), followed by 4 years of subspecialty training.

Candidates are eligible to take the subspecialty certifying examination in their relevant field (e.g., Pediatric ID Certifying Examination) after the completion of a combined 6 years of training. Candidates who wish to fast track through residency require approval from the American Board of Pediatrics to take both the general pediatrics and the pediatric subspecialty certifying examinations.

Career Opportunities in Pediatric Infectious Diseases

According to the Pediatric Infectious Diseases Society, two thirds of all board-certified pediatric ID physicians practice in a medical school or university setting. They may see ID patients in the inpatient or outpatient setting, teach residents and medical students, conduct research, or perform a combination of these activities.

Other pediatric ID physicians work at public health agencies including the Centers for Disease Control and Prevention and the National Institutes of Health. In this capacity, the investigate disease outbreaks, educate the public, and provide leadership in the field of infectious diseases epidemiology. ID specialists are also in great demand by pharmaceutical companies. Their expertise permits involvement in many aspects of the development of vaccines and antimicrobial, antiviral, and antifungal agents. Approximately 5% of pediatric ID specialists are engaged in private sector patient care. Some specialists practice exclusively in the office setting whereas others combine outpatient and inpatient care.

Additional information can be obtained from the American Board of Pediatrics (*www.abp.org*) and the Pediatric Infectious Diseases Society (*www.pids.org*).

B Review Questions and Answers

QUESTIONS

1. A 3-year-old girl presents with unilateral eyelid edema and erythema with mild proptosis. Extraocular movements are restricted. Orbital CT scan confirms the diagnosis of orbital cellulitis. What is the most appropriate antibiotic for empiric therapy in this patient?

   A. Tetracycline
   B. Ceftazidime
   C. Ampicillin-sulbactam
   D. Trimethoprim-sulfamethoxazole
   E. Metronidazole

2. An 18-month-old boy awakens with a hoarse voice and a seal-like "barking" cough. He is relatively well appearing. The oxygen saturation is 100% in room air. On examination, he has suprasternal retractions and mild inspiratory stridor. What is the most appropriate management?

   A. Oral dexamethasone (0.6 mg/kg)
   B. Nebulized racemic epinephrine
   C. Endotracheal intubation
   D. Intramuscular ceftriaxone
   E. Helium-oxygen tent

3. A 4-year-old girl presents with a 3-week history of gradual right neck swelling. The mass has minimal tenderness. On examination, there is overlying violaceous discoloration. She has good dentition. The family has a pet dog but no other animals. What is the most likely infectious cause?

   A. Nontuberculous mycobacteria
   B. *Bartonella henselae*
   C. *Staphylococcus aureus*
   D. Group B *Streptococcus*
   E. Anaerobes

4. A previously healthy 2-year-old boy presents with a 2-day history of worsening fever and cough. On examination, there is tachypnea but no grunting or nasal flaring. No rales are appreciated. Chest radiograph reveals a right lower lobe opacity but no pleural effusion. What antibiotic would be most appropriate in the outpatient treatment of this child with pneumonia?

A. Gentamicin

B. Ciprofloxacin

C. Cephalexin (first-generation cephalosporin)

D. Imipenem

E. Amoxicillin

5. A 9-year-old girl was diagnosed with pneumonia and treated with amoxicillin. She remains febrile after 48 hours of therapy. In addition, she complains of pleuritic chest pain. What should be the next step in the evaluation?

A. Nasopharyngeal bacterial culture

B. Transthoracic needle biopsy

C. Mycoplasma polymerase chain reaction of the nasopharyngeal aspirate

D. Chest radiograph

E. Radionuclide milk scan

6. Which of the following is associated with toxic shock syndrome due to *Streptococcus pyogenes*?

A. Epstein-Barr virus infection

B. Tampon use

C. Varicella infection

D. Prolonged hospitalization

E. Stepping on a nail through a rubber-soled sneaker

7. A 12-year-old boy presents to the emergency department with an infected hand wound. *Eikenella corrodens* is isolated from wound culture. What is the most likely mechanism of injury?

A. Shearing sheep

B. Punched brother in the mouth

C. Bitten by dog

D. Lawn mower injury

E. Boating accident

8. A 2-year-old boy presents with a 7-day history of fever to 39.4°C. On examination, he has bilateral nonpurulent conjunctivitis and dry, cracked, peeling lips. His hands and feet are swollen and mildly tender. A desquamating rash appeared on the buttocks and groin area several days after fever onset. Uveitis is detected on ophthalmologic examination. What is the most appropriate management?

A. Treat with gamma globulin regardless of echocardiogram results

B. Treat with high-dose acetaminophen

C. Treat with amoxicillin

D. Defer specific treatment until the fever has been present for at least 10 days

E. Treat with gamma globulin only if echocardiogram is abnormal

9. A 9-day-old infant presents with a temperature of 38.8°C. On examination, he is well appearing. There are no findings of focal bacterial infection. What is the most appropriate treatment of this child?

A. Discharge home to follow-up with the pediatrician the next morning

B. Blood culture, CBC, and empiric antibiotics only if the white blood cell count exceeds 15,000/mm^3

C. CBC, blood culture, and intramuscular ceftriaxone

D. CBC, blood, urine, and CSF cultures, and empiric antibiotics

E. Consult infectious diseases for evaluation of fever of unknown origin

10. An 11-year-old boy residing in Connecticut develops a 10-cm erythematous macular rash with central clearing on his leg. The rash has expanded since 4 days ago when it was only 5 cm in diameter. What is the most appropriate management?

A. Test for Lyme IgM and IgG antibodies

B. Test for Rocky Mountain spotted fever antibodies

C. Prescribe oral doxycycline

D. Send a blood culture and administer intramuscular ceftriaxone

E. Obtain an electrocardiogram

11. What is the most appropriate test to perform on the blood of a neonate born to an HIV-positive mother?

A. HIV antibody by ELISA

B. HIV DNA PCR

C. CD4$^+$ count

D. HIV antibody by Western blot

E. Total WBC count

12. A 2-month-old boy presents to your office for a well-child visit. On examination you detect a harsh holosystolic murmur suggestive of a ventricular septal defect. Chest radiograph reveals a right-sided aortic arch and absence of the thymus. What is the most likely diagnosis?

A. Wiskott-Aldrich syndrome

B. Transient hypogammaglobulinemia of infancy

C. IgA deficiency

D. Chronic granulomatous disease

E. 22Q11.2 deletion syndrome (DiGeorge syndrome)

13. What is the most common mechanism by which bacteria cause osteomyelitis in children?

A. Direct inoculation from surgery

B. Direct inoculation from penetrating trauma

C. Hematogenous seeding after bacteremia

D. Spread from adjacent septic arthritis

E. Spread from adjacent cellulitis

14. Which of the following is considered a HACEK organism?

A. *Haemophilus influenzae* type b

B. *Arcanobacterium haemolyticum*

C. Cytomegalovirus

D. *Escherichia coli*

E. *Kingella* species

15. A 7-year-old girl presents in January with a 1-day history of fever, headache, photophobia, and vomiting. On examination, she is ill appearing. Passive flexion of the neck results in spontaneous flexion of the hips (Brudzinski sign). You suspect bacterial meningitis. Her serum glucose is 70 mg/dL. Which of the following cerebrospinal fluid results is most consistent with bacterial meningitis?

	WBC (per mm^3)	Neutrophils (%)	Protein (mg/dL)	Glucose (mg/dL)
A.	2000	85	90	30
B.	200	50	200	20
C.	200	75	20	55
D.	100	8	20	55
E.	200	30	90	55

16. Which TORCH infection is most commonly associated with *periventricular* intracranial calcifications?

    A. Rubella
    B. Cytomegalovirus
    C. Syphilis
    D. Toxoplasma
    E. Herpes simplex virus

17. A hospitalized patient with which one of the following diseases would require droplet precautions?

    A. *Clostridium difficile* colitis
    B. Influenza
    C. Rotavirus gastroenteritis
    D. Respiratory syncytial virus bronchiolitis
    E. Hepatitis A

18. Which of the following antiviral agents is effective in managing influenza B infections?

    A. Acyclovir
    B. Amantadine
    C. Cidofovir
    D. Oseltamivir
    E. Chicken soup

19. A 12-month-old girl presents for evaluation of fever and abdominal pain. Urinalysis reveals 2+ leukocyte esterase by dipstick. What pathogen will most likely be isolated from urine culture?

    A. *Escherichia coli*
    B. *Staphylococcus aureus*
    C. *Staphylococcus saprophyticus*
    D. *Corynebacterium* species
    E. α-Hemolytic streptococci

20. Seizures are an extraintestinal manifestation of which of the following gastrointestinal pathogens?

A. *Campylobacter jejuni*
B. *Escherichia coli* O157:H7
C. *Yersinia enterocolitica*
D. *Clostridium difficile*
E. *Shigella* species

21. A 4-year-old girl with acute lymphocytic leukemia has been neu-tropenic for 21 days during induction chemotherapy. She now complains of headache and facial pain. On examination, there is left peri-orbital swelling. A small area of blackened eschar is noted within the nose. Sinusitis due to *Aspergillus* species is suspected. What is the most appropriate therapy while awaiting surgical debridement?

A. Fluconazole
B. Voriconazole
C. Nystatin
D. Clotrimazole troches
E. Acyclovir

22. A 6-month-old girl presents with severe hypoxia and tachypnea. On examination there are marked intercostal retractions but few rales. In talking with the mother you discover that the father is HIV positive. The mother has never been tested. This information, combined with the clinical presentation, makes you suspect *Pneumocystis carinii* pneumonia. You order a bronchoscopy. Which of the following tests would be most useful in making the diagnosis?

A. Gomori silver stain
B. Ziehl-Neelsen stain
C. Kirby-Bauer test
D. India ink stain
E. Plate on chocolate agar

23. A 17-year-old boy with a ventriculoperitoneal shunt presents with headache, fever, vomiting, and photophobia. Which of the following organisms is most likely to cause a ventricular shunt infection?

A. *Streptococcus pneumoniae*
B. *Citrobacter diversus*
C. Group B *Streptococcus*
D. *Streptococcus milleri* group
E. *Staphylococcus epidermidis*

24. A 2-year-old child is evaluated in the infectious diseases clinic for recurring "boils." What is the medical term for "boil"?

A. Bordet-Gengou
B. Shell vial
C. Furuncle
D. Tache noir
E. Bubo

25. A 10-year-old boy presents to the emergency department several hours after eating leftover fried rice at home. He complains of nausea and diarrhea. You suspect food poisoning. What is the most likely organism?

    A. *Bacillus cereus*
    B. *Kingella kingae*
    C. *Cryptosporidium ovale*
    D. *Enterobius vermicularis*
    E. *Clostridium difficile*

ANSWER KEY

1. C	10. C	19. A
2. A	11. B	20. E
3. A	12. E	21. B
4. E	13. C	22. A
5. D	14. E	23. E
6. C	15. A	24. C
7. B	16. B	25. A
8. A	17. B	
9. D	18. D	

ANSWERS

1. **C.** The most likely causes of orbital cellulitis include gram-positive organisms such as *Staphylococcus aureus, Streptococcus pneumoniae,* and *Streptococcus pyogenes,* and anaerobes. The ampicillin component of ampicillin-sulbactam provides excellent coverage against *S. pneumoniae* and *S. pyogenes.* The sulbactam component, a β-lactamase inhibitor, allows the antibiotic to be effective against bacteria that have β-lactamase production as a mechanism of resistance (e.g., *S. aureus* and anaerobes). Tetracycline use would be inappropriate in a toddler when other options exist. Potential side effects of prolonged tetracycline use in a toddler include permanent tooth discoloration, enamel defects, and retardation of bone growth. Ceftazidime does not provide adequate coverage against *S. aureus* or anaerobes. Trimethoprim-sulfamethoxazole (Bactrim) is not active against anaerobes and has poor activity against *S. pneumoniae* and *S. pyogenes.* Metronidazole provides excellent anaerobic coverage but has no activity against gram-positive aerobes such as *S. aureus, S. pneumoniae,* and *S. pyogenes*

2. **A.** In a well-appearing child with croup and increased respiratory effort, oral corticosteroids are appropriate to decrease laryngeal edema. The duration of action of dexamethasone is usually more than 36 hours. While a chest radiograph reveals the "steeple sign" in 50% of children with croup, routine radiography is unnecessary since the diagnosis can easily be made by careful clinical evaluation. Racemic epinephrine is required only for severe or acutely worsening respiratory distress. Children receiving racemic epinephrine require several hours of observation since symptoms

can recur (rebound phenomenon) as the effect of epinephrine abates. Endotracheal intubation is needed with respiratory failure *not* in a well-appearing child who can adequately protect his airway. The cause of croup is typically viral. Parainfluenza viruses are the most common cause. Ceftriaxone would be required if bacterial tracheitis or epiglottitis was suspected. Helium, a low-viscosity gas, improves laminar air flow to decrease mechanical work of breathing when mixed with oxygen. This should be considered in children with severe or moderate and worsening croup.

3. **A. Nontuberculous mycobacteria classically cause a gradually progressing cervical adenitis. The minimal tenderness and overlying violaceous hue are clues to the diagnosis. A tuberculin skin test may show mild (5 to 9 mm) induration. Surgical resection is curative.** *Bartonella henselae,* the etiologic agent of cat-scratch disease, is almost always associated with clear contact with a kitten (usually) or older cat (occasionally). Although transmission through contact with a dog has been reported, such a mode of transmission is highly unlikely. *Staphylococcus aureus* is the most common cause of cervical adenitis. However, the infected node presents acutely rather than subacutely. On examination it is usually extremely tender with overlying cellulitis. Group *B Streptococcus* is associated with adenitis in neonates. Anaerobic cervical adenitis is usually associated with dental infection.

4. **E. The most likely bacterial cause of lobar pneumonia in a toddler is** *Streptococcus pneumoniae.* **While the prevalence of drug-resistant** *S. pneumoniae* **is increasing, failures due to penicillin or amoxicillin as a consequence of resistant** *S. pneumoniae* **pneumonia are uncommon.** Gentamicin provides excellent coverage against gram-negative organisms but provides no coverage against *S. pneumoniae,* the most likely bacterial cause of pneumonia in this child. In addition, in the outpatient setting, an oral rather than intravenous antibiotic would be preferred. Oral gentamicin is poorly absorbed and should not be used to manage systemic infection. Ciprofloxacin would be inappropriate in a patient this young when other convenient options are available. First-generation cephalosporins have only fair activity against *S. pneumoniae,* the most likely bacterial cause of pneumonia in young children. Imipenem is effective in management of *S. pneumoniae* but is *not* currently available in an oral formulation. Furthermore, the broad-spectrum coverage provided by imipenem is not required in an otherwise healthy, relatively well-appearing patient with uncomplicated community-acquired pneumonia.

5. **D. In a child with fever and pleuritic chest pain, the most likely diagnosis is pleural effusion complicating pneumonia. A chest radiograph would provide the diagnosis. A blood culture should also be obtained because 10% to 25% of children with pleural effusion have associated bacteremia.** Nasopharyngeal bacterial

cultures correlate poorly with results of lung biopsy and, therefore, are not used in the evaluation of children with pneumonia. Transthoracic needle biopsy should be considered in children with pneumonia who are immunodeficient or clinically worsening without apparent cause. This would not be part of the *initial* evaluation. *Mycoplasma* PCR is useful in diagnosing pneumonia due to *Mycoplasma pneumoniae*. While the diagnosis of *Mycoplasma* infection would explain the poor response to amoxicillin, this is not the first study to consider in a child with fever and pleuritic chest pain. A radionuclide milk scan is useful in diagnosing aspiration in a patient with a history suggestive of aspiration pneumonia or recurrent wheezing. Gastroesophageal reflux would not explain the relatively acute development of fever and pleuritic chest pain in this child.

6. **C. Varicella is associated with invasive infections due to *Streptococcus pyogenes* (group A *Streptococcus*). Varicella vaccine use has decreased the incidence of severe varicella infections by 95%.** Epstein-Barr virus causes an exudative pharyngitis that can be mistaken for "Strep throat." Tampon use is associated with *Staphylococcus aureus* toxic shock syndrome. Prolonged hospitalization is associated with many different types of nosocomial infections, usually due to coagulase-negative staphylococci or aerobic gram-negative rods. Stepping on a nail through a rubber-soled sneaker is associated with *Pseudomonas aeruginosa* osteomyelitis of the foot

7. **B. *Eikenella corrodens* is part of the oral flora of humans. This organism may complicate human bite wounds. A hand injury sustained while punching someone in the mouth is equivalent to a human bite.** The cutaneous form of anthrax can be contracted while working with infected livestock. Inhalational anthrax was known as wool sorter's disease because it often occurred among workers handling infected hides and wool. Dog bite infections can be caused by *Pasteurella* species and *Capnocytophaga* species. Lawn mower injuries can be complicated by infection with organisms from the skin or soil, including staphylococci, *Escherichia coli*, *Aeromonas hydrophila*, *Stenotrophomonas maltophilia*, *Pseudomonas* species, *Enterobacter* species, and *Clostridium tetani*. In injuries or bites occurring in marine environments, consider *Vibrio* species, *Aeromonas hydrophila*, *Plesiomonas shigelloides*, and *Pseudomonas* species.

8. **A. This child has Kawasaki syndrome. Treatment with gamma globulin within 10 days of symptom onset reduces the incidence of coronary aneurysms in Kawasaki syndrome from 15%–25% to 5%.** High-dose *aspirin* NOT acetaminophen is used in the management of Kawasaki. Amoxicillin is used to manage scarlet fever, an infection caused by group A *Streptococcus*. Scarlet fever is often included in the differential diagnosis of children with Kawasaki syndrome. However, while uveitis is seen in up to 80% of children with

Kawasaki syndrome, it is not associated with scarlet fever. Management of Kawasaki should occur *prior* to the 10th day of fever to reduce the risk of coronary aneurysms. A normal echocardiogram does not exclude the diagnosis of Kawasaki syndrome because not all patients with known Kawasaki develop coronary aneurysms. Furthermore, the initial echocardiogram is *often* normal since aneurysms, when they occur, do not usually develop until 10 to 21 days after symptom onset.

9. **D. Up to 15% of neonates (younger than 30 days) with fever in excess of 38.0°C have a serious bacterial infection, including meningitis, pyelonephritis, and bacteremia. Approximately 65% of neonates with a serious bacterial infection have a normal examination at presentation. This finding has given rise to the saying, "Never trust a baby." Therefore, *all* febrile neonates deserve aggressive evaluation for bacterial infection. This evaluation includes cultures of blood, urine, and CSF. Empiric antibiotics (usually ampicillin plus gentamicin or ampicillin plus cefotaxime) are administered until cultures are negative for at least 48 hours. For a positive culture, treatment is modified as appropriate.** Febrile *infants (ages 2 to 24 months, or 3 to 36 months)* at risk for occult bacteremia may be treated with close follow-up alone if the examination is normal. An alternative acceptable strategy in infants (not neonates) is to selectively administer empiric antibiotics to those at highest risk of occult bacteremia and its complications (such as those with peripheral WBC counts in excess of 15,000/mm^3). The above patient is too young for either of these strategies. *All* febrile neonates require aggressive evaluation, including lumbar puncture, to detect serious bacterial infection. Fever of unknown origin is used to describe a child with more than 2 weeks of fever and an unclear source after careful history, examination, and initial evaluation. This neonate does not meet the criteria for fever of unknown origin.

10. **C. The rash is classic for the erythema migrans rash seen with Lyme disease. Untreated, the rash may gradually expand to 15 to 30 cm in diameter; hence the name "migrans." The appropriate treatment for this early localized stage of Lyme disease is doxycycline. In younger children, amoxicillin can be used. Typical duration of treatment is 14 to 21 days.** When the rash has such a classic appearance, confirmatory antibody studies are not required. Furthermore, early in the course of Lyme disease, antibody studies may be negative. The rash seen in Rocky Mountain spotted fever begins on the extremities and migrates centrally. The rash is typically macular progressing to petechial. Blood culture and empiric ceftriaxone would be reasonable *if* this were a petechial or purpuric rash, raising concern for meningococcemia. An electrocardiogram detects atrioventricular heart block, a complication of early *disseminated* (stage 2) Lyme disease. Since there is only a solitary lesion, this

child has early localized Lyme disease and electrocardiogram will likely be normal (and unnecessary).

11. **B. The HIV DNA PCR is highly sensitive and specific. A positive test should still be repeated to confirm the diagnosis. Infants born to HIV-positive mothers should receive zidovudine for the first 6 weeks of life to decrease the risk of perinatal transmission.** *Pneumocystis carinii* prophylaxis with trimethoprim-sulfamethoxazole should be started at approximately 6 weeks of life and can be discontinued at 4 months if the HIV DNA PCR result remains negative. The HIV ELISA is an IgG-based test. Infants born to HIV-positive mothers have detectable HIV antibodies from intrapartum transmission. This reflects the HIV status of the mother not the infant. The passively acquired antibodies may persist until 15 to 18 months of age in uninfected infants. The $CD4^+$ count is normal in most HIV-infected neonates. This test would not detect the majority of infected neonates. The HIV Western blot test is used to confirm a positive ELISA. Since this is also an IgG antibody–based test, this infant will have detectable antibodies from passive maternal transfer during the third trimester. Antibodies detected in an infant this young reflect the HIV status of the mother, not the infant. The total WBC count is usually normal in HIV-infected neonates. This would not help distinguish infected from uninfected neonates.

12. **E. DiGeorge syndrome is due to defective embryologic development of the third and fourth pharyngeal pouches. Affected children have variable deletions of chromosome 22q11. The thymus is usually hypoplastic or absent. Associated cardiac defects include conotruncal defects, atrial and ventricular septal defects, and aortic arch abnormalities. Other associated defects include palatal insufficiency, esophageal atresia, and bifid uvula.** Wiskott-Aldrich syndrome is associated with the triad of immunodeficiency, eczema, and thrombocytopenia. Transient hypogammaglobulinemia of infancy is an abnormal delay in the onset of antibody production. It is not associated with cardiac defects. IgA deficiency is the most common antibody deficiency with a prevalence of 1 in 400. In most children infection is asymptomatic. Some children present with recurrent sinopulmonary infections. Children with chronic granulomatous disease develop recurrent skin and soft-tissue infections or more invasive infections (e.g., pneumonia, osteomyelitis) with catalase-positive organisms such as *Staphylococcus aureus*.

13. **C. Acute hematogenous osteomyelitis, as the name implies, results from hematogenous seeding following bacteremia. In otherwise healthy children, this is the most common mechanism.** Direct inoculation of bacteria following surgery or penetrating trauma occurs less commonly in children. Extension of cellulitis into the bone is rare. In infants, osteomyelitis may extend into the joint to cause a secondary septic arthritis but septic arthritis rarely extends into the bone to cause osteomyelitis.

14. **E.** The HACEK organisms are oral gram-negative bacilli that cause up to 10% of cases of native valve endocarditis. The acronym HACEK represents the following organisms: *Haemophilus* species (*H. parainfluenzae, H. aphrophilus,* and *H. paraphrophilus*), *Actinobacillus actinomycetemcomitans, Cardiobacterium hominis, Eikenella corrodens,* and *Kingella* species. These organisms have specific nutritional requirements and, as a result, grow slowly in routine culture medium. Therefore, when endocarditis is suspected, blood cultures should be retained for at least 2 weeks to allow for growth of a HACEK organism. These organisms are best treated with a third-generation cephalosporin. *H. influenzae* type b (HIB) was formerly a common cause of childhood meningitis. With the introduction of routine HIB, this organism rarely causes invasive infection in immunized populations. *A. haemolyticum* causes pharyngitis associated with a scarlatiniform rash on the extensor surfaces of the arms and legs. Cytomegalovirus is associated with congenital infections and infectious mononucleosis; in addition, in immunocompromised patients, pneumonia. *E. coli,* a gram-negative rod, causes many different types of infections including urinary tract infections, neonatal meningitis, and catheter-related bloodstream infections. It does not have fastidious growth requirements.

15. **A.** The CSF findings in bacterial meningitis vary depending on the infecting organism as well as the timing of the lumbar puncture in relation to onset of symptoms. Bacterial meningitis is usually associated with dramatic neutrophilic CSF pleocytosis. The protein content is high due to leptomeningeal inflammation while the glucose content is low (less than two thirds the serum level). Tuberculous meningitis presents with a mild pleocytosis but a dramatically elevated protein and low glucose. Children may have associated miliary disease. Viral meningitis (often enteroviruses in the summer) may have a neutrophil predominance early in the illness. As the illness progresses, a lymphocyte predominance develops. The protein may be normal or mildly elevated but the glucose is normal. Lyme meningitis typically presents with a prolonged period of symptoms (often up to 2 weeks). Similar to enteroviruses, Lyme meningitis is most common during the summer months. The pleocytosis is mild and usually mononuclear (many lymphocytes and monocytes but few neutrophils). Herpes simplex virus meningoencephalitis may have a mild-moderate pleocytosis with a dramatically elevated protein. Children may present with confusion and focal seizures, reflecting temporal lobe involvement.

16. **B.** Cytomegalovirus is often associated with periventricular calcifications. It is also the leading cause of sensorineural hearing loss in children. Features of congenital rubella include microcephaly, cataracts, deafness, cardiac defects, hepatosplenomegaly, and "blueberry muffin" rash (represents extramedullary hematopoiesis). Congenital syphilis may manifest as low birth weight, failure to

thrive, hydrocephalus, mucocutaneous bullous lesions, bloody rhinitis ("snuffles"), hepatosplenomegaly, osteochondritis, and jaundice. Infants with toxoplasmosis also have intracranial calcifications. However, in these infants the calcifications tend to be *generalized* rather than periventricular. Herpes simplex virus usually causes a perinatal rather than congenital infection. Vesicular skin lesions are characteristic. Despite prompt initiation of acyclovir, mortality remains high in those with systemic dissemination. Survivors of central nervous system infection have significant neurologic sequelae.

17. **B. Droplet precautions are required for infections spread by propulsion of larger droplets directly onto mucosal surfaces (e.g., conjunctivae, mouth) over a short distance. Influenza is the only one of the choices spread by this route. Other infections requiring droplet precautions in hospitalized patients include pertussis, meningococcemia, rubella, and mycoplasma.** The remaining choices all require contact precautions.

18. **D. Both oseltamivir (Tamiflu) and zanamivir (Relenza) specifically target the neuraminidase protein common to influenza A and B viruses. They ultimately interfere with disaggregation and release of viral progeny. Oseltamivir is administered orally. Zanamivir is delivered to the respiratory tract by oral inhalation. When started within 36 hours of illness, these compounds reduce the duration of illness by 1 to 2 days. Perhaps more importantly, prophylactic administration can prevent influenza in exposed contacts.** Acyclovir has activity against herpes simplex virus, varicella, and, to a lesser extent, Epstein-Barr virus. Amantadine, like rimantadine, is effective against influenza A but *not* influenza B. Cidofovir has activity against adenovirus, cytomegalovirus, Epstein-Barr virus, herpes simplex virus, varicella, and, potentially, smallpox. Technically not an antiviral agent but I won't argue with a grandmother on this one.

19. **A.** *Escherichia coli* **accounts for 70% to 90% of urinary tract infections in young children.** *Staphylococcus aureus* rarely causes isolated urinary tract infections in children. Typically, children with *S. aureus* urinary tract infections have an indwelling urinary catheter predisposing to infection. Otherwise, these children have an additional site of infection such as a renal parenchymal abscess or osteomyelitis. *Staphylococcus saprophyticus* more typically causes urinary tract infections in female *adolescents*. *Corynebacterium* species colonize the periurethra and are usually contaminants. α-Hemolytic streptococci also colonize the periurethra and are usually contaminants.

20. **E. Seizures may precede the bloody diarrhea in children with** *Shigella* **infection, making the diagnosis difficult at first.** *Campylobacter* infections are associated with reactive arthritis, erythema nodosum, and Guillain-Barré syndrome. *Escherichia coli* 0157:H7 is associated with hemolytic uremic syndrome. *Yersinia enterocolitica* is associated with erythema nodosum, glomerulonephritis, and

reactive arthritis. *Clostridium difficile* infections may cause a reactive arthritis.

21. **B. Voriconazole, a triazole antifungal agent, is effective against many fungi, including *Aspergillus* species. The blackened eschar in the nose is a clue to the diagnosis of *Aspergillus* in this immuno-compromised patient.** Fluconazole has activity against several *Candida* species. However, it does not have activity against *Aspergillus* species. Nystatin is useful for oral management of thrush and topical management of candidal dermatitis. It is not effective against *Aspergillus* species. Sinusitis due to *Aspergillus* is life threatening. Appropriate systemic therapy (not a troche) is warranted. Furthermore, clotrimazole has no activity against *Aspergillus*. Acyclovir is effective in the management of viral infections such as those due to herpes simplex and varicella viruses. It does not have antifungal activity.

22. **A. The Gomori silver stain is used to detect *P. carinii*. Other potential stains to detect *P. carinii* include the Giemsa stain and fluorescein-labeled antibody stains.** Ziehl-Neelsen stains detect *Mycobacterium*. The Kirby-Bauer is a disk diffusion test used to determine the susceptibility of bacteria to different antibiotics. To perform the test commercially prepared filter paper disks impregnated with a specified concentration of an antibiotic are applied to the surface of an agar medium inoculated with organism. The antibiotic diffuses into agar and creates a gradient; no growth indicates inhibition. The India ink stain detects *Cryptococcus neoformans,* a cause of pneumonia and meningitis in immunocompromised patients. Chocolate agar contains a nutrient-rich medium that is used to detect *Haemophilus* spp., *Neisseria gonorrhoeae,* and *Neisseria meningitidis*.

23. **E. *Staphylococcus epidermidis* is the most common cause of ventricular shunt–related infections.** *Propionibacterium acnes* and *Staphylococcus aureus* are sometimes isolated. Management includes externalization of the shunt and empiric treatment with broad-spectrum antibiotics. If the organism is identified as *S. epidermidis,* vancomycin alone may be used. Intrathecal vancomycin or oral rifampin is sometimes added for particularly difficult-to-clear infections. Although *Streptococcus pneumoniae* is the most common bacterial cause of meningitis in older children, the rate of infection is not higher in children with ventricular shunt infections. *Citrobacter diversus* is associated with brain abscesses, particularly in neonates. Group B *Streptococcus* causes meningitis and other invasive infections in neonates. It is not typically associated with ventricular shunt infections in older children. Bacteria of the *Streptococcus milleri* group are associated with intracranial complications of sinusitis.

24. **C. The word "boil" is the lay term for furuncle, a bacterial infection of the hair follicle.** Bordet-Gengou is the culture medium for growing *Bordetella pertussis*. The shell vial assay is performed by inoculating

specimens onto cell monolayers using centrifugation. Viral growth in the cell monolayers is then detected using fluorescein-labeled monoclonal antibodies to specific viral antigens. This is an excellent way to culture cytomegalovirus. The tache noir is a necrotic eschar that occurs in patients with rickettsial infections. It originates at the site of the bite and is detected in 30% to 90% of patients. Look for this in the scalp with associated regional lymphadenopathy. Bubo refers to the painful lymphadenopathy in patients with the bubonic plague that develops concurrently in the extremity bitten by flea. After an incubation period of 2 to 10 days, the infected patient develops acute onset of high fever, malaise, myalgias, headache, nausea, and vomiting. The bubo is accompanied by skin lesions in surrounding lymphatic drainage area.

25. **A.** The timing of the illness suggests ingestion of preformed toxin. *Bacillus cereus* is classically associated with fried rice. Typically incubation periods for food-borne illnesses are as follows: less than 6 hours (preformed toxin: *Staphylococcus aureus, Bacillus cereus*); 8 to 16 hours (*Clostridium perfringens, B. cereus*); 16 to 96 hours (*Shigella, Salmonella, Vibrio* spp., invasive *Escherichia coli, Campylobacter jejuni, Yersinia enterocolitica,* caliciviruses). Kingella kingae is associated with arthritis and endocarditis. *Cryptosporidium ovale* causes diarrhea in immunocompromised patients, especially those with HIV infection. *Enterobius vermicularis* is also known as pinworm. It usually causes perineal pruritis and occasionally causes abdominal pain. It can be detected by placing cellophane tape ("Scotch tape" test) around the perineum and then examining the tape under the microscope. It does not typically cause diarrhea. *Clostridium difficile* usually causes diarrhea or colitis in association with broad-spectrum antibiotic use.

C Commonly Prescribed Oral Medications

Note: See alternative source for dosing in neonates. Dosing may vary by indication; check alternative source (e.g., *Physicians' Desk Reference*) to confirm dosing and view information on side effects, drug interactions, and contraindications.

Acyclovir[a]	Mucocutaneous HSV: 1200 mg/m^2/d divided TID × 7–10 days; varicella: 80 mg/kg/d divided QID × 5 d (max. 3200 mg/d)
Albendazole	For many intestinal nematodes, including pinworm: 200 mg (if age >1 but <2 years) or 400 mg (if ≥2 years) as a single dose
Amoxicillin[a]	Standard dose: 20–40 mg/kg/d divided TID; "High-dose": 80–90 mg/kg/d divided TID; adults 250–500 mg TID (max. 3 g/d); endocarditis prophylaxis 50 mg/kg (max. 2 g) 1 h before procedure
Amoxicillin-clavulanate[a]	Dosing based on amoxicillin component. To avoid excessive adverse GI events, use amoxicillin 600 mg/clavulanic potassium 42.9 mg per 5 mL formulation (ES-600) if the dose of clavulanic acid exceeds 10 mg/kg/d using the regular-strength formulation
Azithromycin[a]	Most infections: 10 mg/kg (max. 500 mg) on day 1, then 5 mg/kg/d QD (max. 250 mg) days 2–5; uncomplicated chlamydial cervicitis: 10 mg/kg as single dose (max. 1 g)
Ceftibuten[a]	9 mg/kg/d once each day; adults 400 mg QD (max. 400 mg/d)
Cephalexin[a]	50–100 mg/kg/d divided QID; adults 250–500 mg QID (max. 2 g/d)
Ciprofloxacin[a]	20–30 mg/kg/d divided BID; adults 250–750 mg BID (max. 1.5 g/d)
Clarithromycin[a]	7.5–15 mg/kg/d divided BID; adults 250–500 mg BID (max. 1 g/d); endocarditis prophylaxis: 15 mg/kg (max. 500 mg) 1 h before procedure (use for penicillin-allergic patients)
Clindamycin[b]	15–25 mg/kg/d divided TID; adults 150–450 mg TID (max. 1.8 g/d)
Dicloxacillin	25–50 mg/kg/d divided QID; adults125–500 mg QID (max. 2 g/d)
Doxycycline	4 mg/kg/d divided BID; adults 100 mg BID (max. 200 mg/d)
Erythromycin	30–50 mg/kg/d as base or ethylsuccinate divided TID or QID; adults 250–500 BID-QID as base or 400–800 mg BID-QID as ethylsuccinate (max. 2 g/d)
Isoniazid	Treatment: 10–20 mg/kg/d in 1–2 divided doses; adults 5 mg/kg/d once each day (max. 300 mg/d)

Levofloxacin [a]	Adults 250–750 mg once daily
Mebendazole	Pinworm: 100 mg initially and repeated 2 weeks later
Metronidazole [b]	*Giardia:* 15 mg/kg/d divided TID; *Clostridium difficile* infections 20 mg/kg/d divided QID; adults 250–500 mg QID
Nitazoxanide [c]	Ages 12–47 months: 100 mg BID; ≥4 to 11 years: 200 mg BID; Adolescents and adults 500 mg BID
Paromomycin	25–30 mg/kg/d divided TID (max. 3 g/d)
Penicillin V potassium	15–50 mg/kg/d divided TID or QID; children >12 years and adults 125–500 mg TID or QID (max. 3 g/d)
Rifampin	Meningococcal prophylaxis: 20 mg/kg/d divided BID × 2 days; adults 600 mg BID × 2 days (max. 1200 mg/d)
Tetracycline [a]	20–40 mg/kg/d divided QID; adults 250–500 mg BID to QID (max. 2 g/d)
Trimethoprim-sulfamethoxazole [a] (dosing based on trimethoprim component)	Mild-moderate infections: 6–12 mg TMP/kg/d divided BID; serious infections: 20 mg TMP/kg/d divided BID; adults 1 double-strength tablet (160 mg TMP) BID (max. 320 mg TMP/d)

[a]Requires dose modification in renal impairment.
[b]Requires dose modification in hepatic impairment.
[c]Use with caution in renal or hepatic impairment since specific dosing information not available for these situations.

Suggested Additional Reading

CHAPTER 3

Henry NK, Hoecker JL, Rhodes KH. Antimicrobial therapy for infants and children: guidelines for the inpatient and outpatient practice of pediatric infectious diseases. *Mayo Clin Proc* 2000;75:86–97.

Leclercq R. Mechanisms of resistance to macrolides and lincosamides: nature of the resistance elements and their clinical implications. *Clin Infect Dis* 2002;34:482–492.

Long SS, Dowell SF. Principles of anti-infective therapy. In: Long SS, Pickering LK, Prober CG, eds. *Principles and Practice of Pediatric Infectious Diseases*, 2nd ed. New York: Churchill Livingstone, 2003:1422–1432.

Lustar I, McCracken GH Jr, Friedland IR. Antibiotic pharmacodynamics in the cerebrospinal fluid. *Clin Infect Dis* 1998;27: 1117–1129.

Whitney CG, Farley MM, Hadler J, et al. Increasing prevalence of multidrug-resistant *Streptococcus pneumoniae* in the United States. *N Engl J Med* 2000;343:1917–1924.

CHAPTER 6

Endophthalmitis Vitrectomy Study Group. Results of the Endophthalmitis Vitrectomy Study: a randomized trial of immediate vitrectomy and of intravenous antibiotic for the treatment of postoperative bacterial endophthalmitis. *Arch Ophthalmol* 1995;113:1479–1496.

Jackson WB. Differentiating conjunctivitis of diverse origins. *Surv Ophthalmol* 1993;38:91–104.

Lessner A, Stern GA. Preseptal and orbital cellulitis. *Infect Dis Clin North Am* 1992;6:933–952.

O'Hara, MA. Ophthalmia neonatorum. *Pediatr Clin North Am* 1993;40:715–725.

Shah SS, Gallagher PG. Complications of conjunctivitis due to *Pseudomonas aeruginosa* in a newborn intensive care unit. *Pediatr Infect Dis J* 1998;17:97–102.

CHAPTER 7

Auletta JJ, Chandy CC. Spinal epidural abscesses in children: a 15-year experience and review of the literature. *Clin Infect Dis* 2001;32:9–16.

Mathisen GE, Johnson JP. Brain abscess. *Clin Infect Dis* 1997;25: 763–779.

Saez-Lorenz X, McCracken GH, Jr. Bacterial meningitis in children. *Lancet* 2003;361:2139–2148.

Whitley RJ, Gnann JW. Viral encephalitis: familiar infections and emerging pathogens. *Lancet* 2003;359:507–513.

CHAPTER 8

American Academy of Pediatrics, Subcommittee on Management of Sinusitis and Committee on Quality Improvement. Clinical Practice Guideline: Management of sinusitis. *Pediatrics* 2001; 108:798–808.

Ausejo M, Saenz A, Pham B, et al. The effectiveness of glucocorticoids in treating croup: meta-analysis. *BMJ* 1999;319: 595–600.

Bisno AL, Gerber MA, Gwaltney JM, et al. Diagnosis and management of group A streptococcal pharyngitis: a practice guideline. *Clin Infect Dis* 1997;25:574–583.

Bojrab D, Bruderly T, Abdulrazzak Y. Otitis externa. *Otolaryngol Clin North Am* 1996;29:761–782.

Broughton RA. Non-surgical management of deep neck infections in children. *Pediatr Infect Dis J* 1992;11:14–18.

Ghaffar FA, Wordemann M, McCracken GH. Acute mastoiditis in children: a seventeen-year experience in Dallas, Texas. *Pediatr Infect Dis J* 2001;20:376–380.

Hughes E, Lee JH. Otitis externa. *Pediatr Rev* 2001;22:191–197.

Malhotra A, Krilov LR. Viral croup. *Pediatr Rev* 2001;22:5–12.

CHAPTER 9

Freij BJ, Kusmiesz H, Nelson JD, McCracken GH Jr. Parapneumonic effusions and empyema in hospitalized children: a retrospective review of 227 cases. *Pediatr Infect Dis J* 1984;3: 578–591.

Garrison MM, Christakis DA, Harvey E, Cummings P, Davis RL. Systemic corticosteroids in infant bronchiolitis: a meta-analysis. *Pediatrics* 2000;105:e44.

Ramnath RR, Heller RM, Ben-Ami T, et al. Implications of early sonographic evaluation of parapneumonic effusions in children with pneumonia. *Pediatrics* 1998;101:68–71.

Shah SS, Alpern ER, Zwerling L, McGowan KL, Bell LM. Risk of bacteremia in young children with pneumonia treated as outpatients. *Arch Pediatr Adolesc Med* 2003;157:389–392.

CHAPTER 10

Baltimore RS. Infective endocarditis. In: Jenson HB, Baltimore RS, eds. *Pediatric infectious diseases: principles and practice*, 2nd ed. Philadelphia, WB Saunders, 2002.

Drucker NA, Newberger JW. Viral myocarditis: diagnosis and management. *Adv Pediatr* 1997;44:141–171.

Feldman WE. Bacterial etiology and mortality of purulent pericarditis in pediatric patients: a review of 162 cases. *Am J Dis Child* 1979:133:641.

Ferrieri P, Gewitz MH, Gerber MA, et al. Unique features of infective endocarditis in childhood. *Pediatrics* 2002:109; 931–943.

CHAPTER 11

Altschuler S, Liacouras C, eds. *Clinical pediatric gastroenterology*. New York: Churchill Livingstone, 1998.

Suchy F, Sokol R, Balistreri W, ed. *Liver disease in children*, 2nd ed. Philadelphia: Lippincott Williams & Wilkins, 2001

McEvoy C, Suchy F. Biliary tract disease in children. *Pediatr Clin North Am* 1996;43:75.

Narkewicz M. Biliary atresia; an update on our understanding of the disorder. *Curr Opin Pediatr* 2001;13:435–440.

Committee on Infectious Diseases. *Red Book 2003. Report of the Committee on Infectious Diseases*, 26th ed. Elk Grove Village, IL: American Academy of Pediatrics, 2003.

Schaefer F. Management of peritonitis in children receiving chronic peritoneal dialysis. *Paediatr Drugs* 2003;5:315–325.

CHAPTER 12

American Academy of Pediatrics. Guidelines for the evaluation of sexual abuse of children. *Pediatrics* 1999;103:186–191.

American Academy of Pediatrics. Practice parameter: the diagnosis, treatment, and evaluation of the initial urinary tract infection in febrile infants and young children. *Pediatrics* 1999;103:843–852.

Hoberman A, Wald ER, Hickey RW, et al. Oral versus initial intravenous therapy for urinary tract infections in young febrile children. *Pediatrics* 1999;104:79–86.

Lohr JA, O'Hara SM. Renal (intrarenal and perinephric) abscess. In: Long SS, Pickering LK, Prober CG, eds. *Principles and practice of pediatric infectious diseases*, 2nd edition. New York: Churchill Livingstone: 2003:329–333.

Seigel RM, Schubert CJ, Meyers PA, Shapiro RA. Prevalence of sexually transmitted diseases in children and adolescents evaluated for sexual abuse in Cincinnati: rationale for limited STD testing in prepubertal girls. *Pediatrics* 1995;96:1090–1094.

CHAPTER 13

Bhumbra N, McCullough S. Skin and subcutaneous infections. *Primary Care: Clin Office Pract* 2003;30:1–24.

Rhody C. Bacterial infections of the skin. *Primary Care: Clin Office Pract* 2000;27:459–473.

Stulberg DL, Penrod MA, Blatny RA. Caring for common skin conditions: common bacterial skin infection. *Am Fam Phys* 2002;66:119–124.

Valeriano-Marcet J, Carter J, Vasey F. Soft tissue disease. *Rheum Dis Clin North Am* 2003;29:77–88.

CHAPTER 14

Fernandez M, Carrol CL, Baker CJ. Discitis and vertebral osteomyelitis in children: an 18- year review. *Pediatrics* 2000;105: 1299–1304.

Glazer P, Hu SS. Pediatric spinal infections. *Orthopedic Clin N Am* 1996;27:111–123.

Sonnen GM, Henry NK. Pediatric bone and joint infections. *Pediatr Clin N Am* 1996;43:933–947.

CHAPTER 15

Giroir BT. Recombinant human activated protein C for the treatment of severe sepsis: is there a role in pediatrics? *Curr Opin Pediatr* 2003;15:92–96.

Klein JO. Management of the febrile child without a focus of infection in the era of universal pneumococcal immunization. *Pediatr Infect Dis J* 2002;21:584–588.

Mermel LA, Farr BM, Sherertz RJ, Raad II, O'Grady N, Harris JS. Guidelines for the management of intravascular catheter-related infections. *Clin Infect Dis* 2001;32:1249–1272.

CHAPTER 16

Appelgren P, Bjornhagen V, Bragderyd K, Jonsson CE, Ransjo U. A prospective study of infections in burn patients. *Burns* 2002;28:39–46.

Bell LM, Baker MD, Beatty D, Taylor L. Infections in severely traumatized children. *J Pediatr Surg.* 1992;27:1394–1398.

Cummings P. Antibiotics to prevent infection in patients with dog bite wounds: a meta-analysis of randomized trials. *Ann Emerg Med* 1994;23:535–540.

Hollander JE. Singer AJ. Laceration management *Ann Emerg Med* 1999;34:356–367.

Talan DA, Citron DM, Abrahamian FM, Moran GJ, Goldstein EJ. Bacteriologic analysis of infected dog and cat bites. *N Engl J Med* 1999;340:85–92.

CHAPTER 17

Arav-Boger R, Pass RF. Diagnosis and management of cytomegalovirus infection in the newborn. *Pediatr Ann* 2002;31:719–724.

Cooper LZ, Alford CA Jr. Rubella. In: Remington JS, Klein JO, eds. *Infectious diseases of the fetus and newborn infant*, 5th ed. Philadelphia: WB Saunders, 2001:347–388.

Correa AG. Congenital syphilis: evaluation, diagnosis, and treatment. *Semin Pediatr Infect Dis* 1994;4:30–34.

Kimberlin DW, Lin C-Y, Jacobs RF, et al. Natural history of neonatal herpes simplex virus infections in the acyclovir era. *Pediatrics* 2001;108:223–229.

Remington JS, McLeod R, Thulliez P, Desmonts G. Toxoplasmosis. In: Remington JS, Klein JO, eds. *Infectious diseases of the fetus and newborn infant*, 5th ed. Philadelphia: WB Saunders, 2001:205–346.

CHAPTER 18

Alpern ER, Alessandrini EA, Bell LM, Shaw KN, McGowan KL. Occult bacteremia from a pediatric emergency department:

current prevalence, time to detection, and outcome. *Pediatrics* 2000;106:505–511.

Baker MD, Bell LM, Avner JR. Outpatient management without antibiotics of fever in selected infants. *N Engl J Med* 1993;329:1437–1441.

Baker MD, Bell LM. Unpredictability of serious bacterial illness in febrile infants from birth to 1 month of age. *Arch Pediatr Adolesc Med* 1999;153:508–511.

Gorelick MH, Shaw KN. Clinical decision rule to identify young febrile children at risk for UTI. *Arch Pediatr Adolesc Med* 2000;154:386–390.

Mason WH, Takashahi M. Kawasaki syndrome. *Clin Infect Dis* 199928:169–187.

Ryan ET, Wilson ME, Kain KC. Illness after international travel. *N Engl J Med* 2002;347:505–516.

Shah SS, Zaoutis TE. Fever following international travel: what's bugging this child? *Pediatr Case Rev* 2003;3:44–46.

CHAPTER 19

Jacobs RF, Schutze GE. Ehrlichiosis in children. *J Pediatr* 1997;131:184–192.

Leach CT. Human herpesvirus 6 and 7 infections in children: agents of roseola and other syndromes. *Curr Opinion Pediatr* 2000;12:269–274.

Mandl KD, Stack AM, Fleisher GR. Incidence of bacteremia in infants and children with fever and petechiae. *J Pediatr* 1997; 131:398–404.

Maslers EJ, Olson GS, Weiner SJ, Paddock CD. Rocky Mountain spotted fever: a clinician's dilemma. *Arch Intern Med* 2003;163:769–774.

Nelson B, Jill S, Stone MS. Update on selected viral exanthems. *Curr Opin Pediatr* 2000;12:359–364.

Rosenstein NE, Perkins BA, Stephens DS, Popovic T, Huges JM. Meningococcal disease. *N Engl J Med* 2001;344:1378-1388..

Steele AC. Medical progress: Lyme disease. *N Engl J Med* 2001;345:115–125.

Wells LC, Smith JC, Weston V, Collier J, Rutter N. The child with a non-blanching rash: how likely is meningococcal disease? *Arch Dis Child* 2001;85:218–222.

CHAPTER 20

Hughes WT, Armstrong D, Bodey GP, et al. 2002 Guidelines for the use of antimicrobial agents in neutropenic patients with cancer. *Clin Infect Dis* 2002;34:730–51.

Neville K, Renbarger J, Dreyer Z. Pneumonia in the immuno-compromised pediatric cancer patient. *Semin Respir Infect* 2002;17:21–32

Shenep JL, Flynn PM, Baker DK, et al. Oral cefixime is similar to continued intravenous antibiotics in the empirical treatment of febrile neutropenic children with cancer. *Clin Infect Dis* 2001;32:36–43.

CHAPTER 21

American Academy of Pediatrics, Committee on Pediatric AIDS. Evaluation and medical treatment of the HIV-exposed infant. *Pediatrics* 1997;99:909–917.

Centers for Disease Control and Prevention. Public Health Service Task Force recommendations for the use of antiretroviral drugs in pregnant women infected with HIV-1 for maternal health and for reducing perinatal HIV-1 transmission in the United States. *MMWR Morb Mortal Wkly Rep* 1998:47 (RR-02). (regular revisions available on line: http://aidsinfo.nih.gov/).

Havens PL, and the Committee on Pediatric AIDS. Postexposure prophylaxis in children and adolescents for nonoccupational exposure to Human Immunodeficiency Virus. *Pediatrics* 2003; 111:1475–1489.

Working Group on Antiretroviral Therapy and Medical Management of HIV-Infected Children. Guidelines for the use of antiretroviral agents in pediatric HIV infection. Updated and available on line: http://aidsinfo.nih.gov/ (revised June 25, 2003).

CHAPTER 23

Burnett MW, Bass JW, Cook BA. Etiology of osteomyelitis complicating sickle cell disease. *Pediatrics* 1998;101:296–297.

Davis PB, Drumm M, Konstan MW. Cystic fibrosis. State of the art. *Am J Respir Crit Care Med* 1996;154;1229–1256.

Fishman JA, Rubin RH. Infection in organ-transplant recipients. *N Engl J Med* 1998;338:1741–1751.

Green M, Michaels MG. Infections in solid organ transplant recipients. In: Long SS, Pickering LK, Prober CG, eds. *Principles and practice of pediatric infectious diseases*, 2nd ed. New York: Churchill Livingstone, 2003:554–561.

Ho M, Miller G, Atchison W, et al. Epstein-Barr virus infections and DNA hybridization studies in post transplantation lymphoma and lymphoproliferative lesions: the role of primary infection. *J Infect Dis* 1985;152:876–886.

Norris CF, Smith-Whitley K, McGowan KL. Positive blood cultures in sickle cell disease: time to positivity and clinical outcome. *J Pediatr Hematol Oncol* 2003;25:390–395.

Schaffner A. Pretransplant evaluation for infections in donors and recipients of solid organs. *Clin Infect Dis* 2001;33(Suppl 1):S9–S14.

Wong WY, Overturf GD, Pwars DR. Infection caused by *Streptococcus pneumoniae* in children with sickle cell disease: epidemiology, immunologic mechanisms, prophylaxis and vaccination. *Clin Infect Dis* 1992;14:1124–1136.

CHAPTER 24

Henretig FM, Cieslak TJ, Eitzen EM. Biological and chemical terrorism. *J Pediatr* 2002;141:311–326.

Patt HA, Feigin RD. Diagnosis and management of suspected cases of bioterrorism: a pediatric perspective. *Pediatrics* 2002; 109:685–692.

Swartz MN. Recognition and management of anthrax: an update. *N Engl J Med* 2001;345:1621–1626.

CHAPTER 25

Bolyard EA, Tablan OC, Williams WW, et al. Guideline for infection control in healthcare personnel. *Infect Control Hosp Epidemiol* 1998;19:407–463.

Committee on Infectious Diseases. *2003 Red Book. Report of the Committee on Infectious Diseases,* 26th ed. Elk Grove Village, IL: American Academy of Pediatrics.

Havens PL and the Committee on Pediatric AIDS. Postexposure Prophylaxis in Children and Adolescents for Nonoccupational Exposure to Human Immunodeficiency Virus. *Pediatrics* 2003; 111:1475–1489.

Index